DEDICATION

Twenty-one years ago, after seeing four doctors but getting no definite diagnosis, I was recommended to a "young, cutting-edge rheumatologist at UCLA"—his name was Kenneth Kalunian. Without hesitation he diagnosed me with rheumatoid arthritis, even though my tests were not conclusive. He led me through my medical journey with hope and the best possible care. He never once gave up on me or my disease. Whatever the problem was, he had an answer, a solution, a hope for the future. Without him this story would not have been possible. How do you say thank you to someone who gives you back your life?

Dr. Ken Kalunian, this book is for you and all the people you help with your incredible medical care and your unwavering dedication to research.

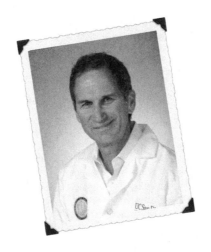

Dr. Ken Kalunian

take me
HOME
from the
OSCARS

ALSO BY CHRISTINE SCHWAB

A Grown-up Girl's Guide to Style

Quickstyle (published under the name Christine Kunzelman)

take me
HOME
from the
OSCARS

Arthritis, Television, Fashion, and Me

CHRISTINE SCHWAB

Skyhorse Publishing

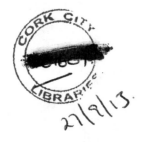

Some names and identifying characteristics have been changed. Some sequences and details of events have been changed.

Copyright © 2011 by Christine Schwab

All Rights Reserved.

No part of this book may be reproduced in any manner without the express written consent of the publisher, except in the case of brief excerpts in critical reviews or articles. All inquiries should be addressed to Skyhorse Publishing, 307 West 36th Street, 11th Floor, New York, NY 10018.

Skyhorse Publishing books may be purchased in bulk at special discounts for sales promotion, corporate gifts, fund-raising, or educational purposes. Special editions can also be created to specifications.
For details, contact the Special Sales Department, Skyhorse Publishing, 307 West 36th Street, 11th Floor, New York, NY 10018 or info@skyhorsepublishing.com.

Skyhorse® and Skyhorse Publishing® are registered trademarks of Skyhorse Publishing, Inc.®, a Delaware corporation.

www.skyhorsepublishing.com

10 9 8 7 6 5 4 3 2 1

Library of Congress Cataloging-in-Publication Data is available on file.
ISBN: 978-1-61608-264-2

Printed in the United States of America

CONTENTS

Foreword

by Deborah Norville

How appropriate that Christine Schwab's very personal book should reference the Oscars. If anyone deserves a gold statuette for "Best Actress," it is she. For virtually all of the more than twenty years that I have known her, I did not know she was putting on an award-winning act. Smiling through the pain, improvising ways to accommodate physical limitations—and all the while terrified someone would discover her secret.

When she wore sneakers with the laces undone, I figured it was just my oh-so-stylish fashionista friend once again at the vanguard of style trends. I thought nothing of the wrap coats. Hands in the pockets during a walking interview on camera? She's just cool. I had no idea it was all part of an elaborate ruse Christine Schwab was orchestrating to keep her disease deeply hidden from everyone except her immediate family and her doctors.

Incredibly, Christine's "secret" was not a terminal illness or a highly contagious disease. It wasn't connected with promiscuous behavior, illicit drugs, or over-indulgence of any sort. But as a television commentator whose beat was fashion, it may as well have been. Christine's shame was she had RA, rheumatoid arthritis. Never mind that RA strikes women in their prime, usually between 30 and 50. Forget the fact that it's an autoimmune disease that is not contagious. Most people don't know and don't care: they hear arthritis and they think "useless gnarled old person." If Christine were to live to be one hundred, that description could never be applied to her.

I will always remember the day I met Christine. How could I not? It was my wedding day and there were two radiant women at the reception. One, of course, was me, the bride—thrilled to have just said "I do" to my best friend and the man of my dreams. The other was this woman I'd never met—the beautiful woman who was glowing while we cut the cake. She was the guest of the man who discovered me when I was in college and gave me my first television opportunity. I knew when my friend Shelly Schwab asked if he could bring a date to our wedding, she must have been someone special. You know, the kind of date who's got 'long term potential.' When I saw them together at the reception, I immediately thought, "I hope you were listening, because you are *definitely* going to be repeating the vows I just said."

In fact Shelly and Christine *did* get married and she and I soon became fast friends. Though she was based in Los Angeles and I was in New York, we saw one another frequently. She'd contribute fashion commentary and expertise to my television show or someone else's or we'd grab lunch when she was in town for the fashion shows or a public appearance. Christine was everything I aspired to be: polished, put together, and endlessly positive. I lived through her exciting stories of life on Hollywood's front lines with Shelly, who by now was a serious power player in the television business. When she wrote her wonderfully accessible books on everyday style, it encouraged me to try putting words down on paper. If there was a "Golden Girl," it was Christine.

But appearances deceive.

Christine's email telling me she'd written another book was no surprise. Of course she'd written another book—the woman's a dynamo. I loved the title: *Take Me Home From the Oscars*. "Oh, goodie," I thought! "A wonderfully dish-y book on life in Hollywood's inner circle. Deals, dinner parties, what the stars are *really* like." Her book will be an instant hit! I was honored when she asked if I would contribute a couple of words of support.

When the manuscript arrived, the subtitle stopped me cold. Rheumatoid arthritis? Christine? It didn't make sense. I began reading and my eyes and heart were opened. Of course I never knew. If all of us live in a youth-oriented society, Christine worked in a youth-obsessed industry. Only a handful of people reach Christine's level of success in television. Given the fickleness of the business, even the slightest hint of something amiss, especially a chronic illness associated with disfigurement, would result in the phone going silent almost overnight. The demand for Christine's expertise would dry up and all those years building a brand as a respected authority on fashion would be for naught.

That's why Christine asked me to write a few words for her book. She knew I understood. I too had battled rheumatoid arthritis, not as a patient, but as the daughter of a woman who bravely battled the disease for more than half the time I had my mom. Diagnosed when I was ten, my mom died of complications of rheumatoid arthritis when I was twenty. My heart broke to think of the physical agony I knew Christine had experienced. I completely understood the fear that rode sidesaddle with her as she looked for medical help. Would the doctors find a treatment that helped? Would her career be over if her disease were "outed"? More chilling, the question she dared not let form: Would Shelly stand by her? It's no secret that three out of four couples dealing with chronic illness get divorced.

Someone once said, "To see your drama clearly is to be liberated from it."

With clarity of vision that can only come from deep introspection, Christine Schwab takes readers on a journey through a life that has certainly been dramatic. From her childhood bouncing among foster homes to the tough years as a young woman trying to make it, it's easy to understand why Christine feared her happy-ever-after ending of the perfect mate and career success would be decimated by RA. Christine's entire life had been punctuated by rejection. Perhaps that cycle hadn't been broken after all?

Ultimately the drama of Christine's RA is liberating, both for her and for the reader. In exquisite prose, she explores the lasting impact of her life experiences and gently encourages us to do the same. Her odyssey through the mysteries of her disease is infuriating, bewildering, yet ultimately inspiring, as her perseverance in demanding the right care results in a treatment that's put her disease in remission. We are all better advocates for ourselves and our families thanks to the lessons shared by Christine.

Finally, Christine shares with us this realization. True love isn't shattered by the vicissitudes of life but rather strengthened by it. St. Paul got it right in his letter to the Corinthians: "Love bearest all things." Indeed, I suspect today if Christine Schwab says, "Take me home from the Oscars," it's not for any reason other than home with her very special husband is the only place she wants to be.

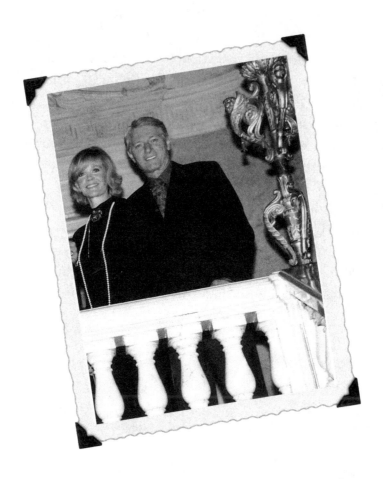

Life in my world didn't get any better than attending the Oscars . . . that is if you can stay for the show.

1

Nobody Walks Out of the
Academy Awards

MARCH 27, 1995

"Welcome to the 67th Annual Academy Awards," the handsome young valet attendant said as he opened the door of our black town car. As he reached in to help me out, I quickly slipped out of my sneakers and into heels. I stepped onto the red carpet, reached for my husband's hand, and took my first deep breath of the fresh spring air that was alive with anticipation of the evening to come.

Thousands of anxious, screaming fans overflowed from the temporary bleachers lining the Boulevard. The thunder of their cheers made the wooden structures sway. Hundreds of paparazzi crowded shoulder-to-shoulder, yelling celebrity names in hopes of getting that one perfect shot.

Producers dressed in their black-on-black event outfits pushed through the crowds, talking on their headsets, confirming which stars had arrived and were ready for live television interviews. Publicists, their worker-bee status obvious from their nonjeweled business attire, scurried behind their celebrities, making sure every hair was in place, each piece of lint removed, before the red-carpet cameras rolled.

The imposing Shrine Auditorium stood at the top of the staircase, waiting for the arrival of the biggest names in entertainment. I wore my new black taffeta Ralph Lauren dress and sheer coat with fabulous chandelier earrings that dusted my shoulders as I walked. Judging from the stares of the crowd, on the outside I looked Oscar worthy. On the inside, the pain pills that I had just managed to swallow as the limo pulled up to the Shrine were attempting to mask my secret inner battle. I had only one goal: Make it through the evening.

It doesn't get much better than the Academy Awards for those of us who work in entertainment, as both my husband and I did. Hollywood boasts dozens of awards shows, but being invited to the Academy Awards is considered the pinnacle of success. Shelly was president of television distribution at Universal Studios. I was a television style reporter, working on *Entertainment Tonight, Oprah, NBC Nightly News,* and *Live with Regis and Kathie Lee.* We had met eight years earlier at the Hollywood Television Executives luncheon at the Beverly Wilshire Hotel, and married three years later, to the day. Life was paradise. Little did we know that over the next seven years a chronic disease would invade my body and try to take it all away from us.

We were truly a power couple. Our social life involved premieres, screenings, political functions, charity events, and glamorous parties. Our business life involved power brokers and celebrities; Shelly worked in back of the camera, I was in front. Given my family roots, it was the least likely place for me to end up.

On this warm March afternoon we walked up the red carpet at the Oscars with hundreds of A-listers. Waiting for the auditorium doors to open, Shelly chatted with Lucy Salhany, president of television at Fox, and David Geffen, who had recently launched DreamWorks with Steven Spielberg and Jeffrey Katzenberg. Geffen defied the traditional tuxedo with his trademark black T-shirt and suit. I remembered thinking he looked like a young man who had crashed the party. Because of the throbbing pain running uncontrollably through my body, I couldn't concentrate on anything they were saying, but that was fine because spouses are almost invisible when executives are together. They didn't notice me shift from foot to foot, trying to find some relief from the pressure of standing on my swollen feet, which by now were bulging out of my designer shoes. Today, because of the unusually hot weather, every woman's feet were most likely hurting, but my pain was from rheumatoid arthritis, a disease that was taking over my body and, unfortunately, my life.

The medical definition of rheumatoid arthritis is an autoimmune disease that causes chronic inflammation of the joints and also other organs. Autoimmune diseases are illnesses that occur when the body's tissues are mistakenly attacked by their own immune system. The immune system contains a complex organization of cells and antibodies designed normally to seek and destroy invaders of the body, particularly infections. The definition that really hit home for me was simply when my doctor said that my immune system was attacking itself, actually eating away at my own bones and joints. Today that was exactly what it felt like. The gnawing made my insides scream with pain each time I made the slightest movement with my feet, or the smallest shift of a leg. A tiny step felt like bits of gravel were grinding against the bones in my feet. Even when I was standing completely still my body ached, but I had to keep my outside together.

Shelly and I sought out a place in the shade even though the celebrity viewing was not as good.

"Shelly, I'm melting," I complained, dabbing at my forehead, trying not to disturb my makeup.

"It's not too bad. Maybe you're just overheated," he said, distracted by all the hoopla.

"Maybe," I replied. I didn't want to let on that I was having one of my bad days. Lately there had been far too many bad days, and

I had decided my husband ought not to have to deal with every one, especially at the Academy Awards.

I continued shifting from one foot to the other, trying to alleviate the throbbing pain that pulsed its way up from my aching feet into my calves and thighs. I couldn't find a comfortable position. Shelly put his arm around my waist to steady me. "Are you okay, Christine?"

"I'll be fine. I took another Percocet for the pain in the car, but it hasn't kicked in."

Shelly lifted the hem of my long skirt. "Ah, your feet are swollen. You should have told me you were having a bad day. Let's sit inside where it's cooler."

"But we'll miss everything," I complained. "Nobody's inside yet."

"No, you're hurting. We're going in," he said, firmly taking my black-lace-gloved hand and supporting me as we entered the almost vacant theater. Frustrated, I looked around at all the empty seats. Nobody took a seat early. Nobody.

"Great seats," Shelly said as we sat down to the left of the stage. Seat fillers were busy removing life-sized pictures of the celebrities whose seats they would fill as stars were called to the stage. Stage managers and directors rushed up and down the aisles checking last-minute details. Tuxedoed cameramen positioned themselves around the aisles, trying to memorize the nominated celebrities' seats so they wouldn't miss any important shots.

Shelly leaned over to give me a kiss. "It's about twenty degrees cooler in here," he said as his lips touched the salty taste of an escaped tear making its way down my cheek. "What's this, you're crying?" he whispered. "Are you all right?"

"I'm fine," I answered, trying to sound calm.

"Why don't you slip off your shoes?"

"I can't. My feet are so swollen I won't be able to get them back on."

I faced forward to prevent him from seeing another tear escape. The tears from pain mixed with frustration and embarrassment continued to roll down my face. I reached for my sunglasses before anyone could notice. The orchestra played the nominated songs as guests began to file in to their seats. Each time someone entered our aisle, we had to stand, fold our seats, and move back as far as possible to make way for the full dresses. Each time I stood the pain shot a little farther up my body. I tried, unsuccessfully, to get comfortable in my chair. Shelly grimaced at me, "Christine, you don't look so good, are you going to be okay? This is a long show."

"I'll be . . ." and then I couldn't talk. I could only dab at the tears. Excruciating pain pierced every crevice of my body. My feet throbbed, begging to be let out of my shoes. The swollen joints in my body felt as if they were trying to break through my skin to find more room. I couldn't sit still. Just the brushing of Shelly's coat sleeve against my arm hurt. Nobody cried at the Oscars unless it was during an acceptance speech.

"Come, on, we're getting out of here," Shelly said, standing up.

"No, please, please sit down," I whispered. "I'll be okay, we can't leave, really, I'll . . ."

But I knew I wouldn't feel better. This was a major flare-up, and I'd had them before. Medication would not control the pain. And so slowly, painfully, reluctantly, I stood. We made our way to the back of the auditorium, the only people walking out as everyone else walked in. Outside we moved out of the way as the frantic last-minute arrivals rushed by. Tom Hanks, the favored best actor winner, was shuffling through the sea of demanding reporters. Annette Bening and Warren Beatty, arm in arm, took my breath away with their elegance as they briskly moved toward the entrance. Clint Eastwood, the elder statesman, parted the sea of people like a modern-day Moses. Nobody noticed that we were walking in the wrong direction. Shelly was busy on his cell phone calling the driver, who had probably just settled into a leisurely lunch at a nearby restaurant with the other drivers, gossiping about which celebrity clients were the biggest jerks. I held my heels in my hands as I left the red carpet and walked on hot asphalt in front of the now empty limo line. The rough pavement tore the feet of my pantyhose. I was relieved, but regret and embarrassment overwhelmed me. We'd come all this way. How could we just go home? What would everyone think when they saw that Shelly Schwab's seat was vacant at the most important event of the year? Would this affect his career? Our marriage? Would my disease ruin what he had built? What we had built together?

"The car will be here in five minutes," Shelly said, snapping his cell phone shut, pleased that he had located the driver. Whatever the situation, Shelly took comfort in being in control. I gathered enough saliva in my mouth to swallow another Percocet for the pain. Surely this one would give me some relief. We both turned and looked at the empty red carpet. Only the bleacher fans, the cameras, and reporters remained. Slowly, the big heavy doors of the Shrine Auditorium closed. I could hear Shelly whispering to the confused driver that yes, we did want him to take us back home.

"I feel bad making you miss the show," I apologized, guilt distracting me from my physical pain, but only for a second. The thought of suggesting Shelly stay without me was out of my realm at the moment. I didn't think I could make it to find the driver and the car without him. Pain and the need to escape this confined environment overtook all of my sensibilities.

"You know it really doesn't matter to me, you're the one who loves these things. I enjoy watching you. We'll be home in time to see most of the show," Shelly assured me.

"What about your colleagues? What will they think seeing you leave the Academy Awards?" Shelly only shrugged and smiled that smile of total confidence.

We drove in cool, quiet comfort, my shoes sitting empty on the floor of the car, my red, swollen feet propped on Shelly's lap, toes sticking through the holes of my ruined stockings. The swelling had made all my toes appear to be glued together, like flesh-colored swim fins. Shelly's strong, gentle hand rested firm and lovingly on my taffeta-covered knee. I couldn't let him know that things were getting worse. How would it look if he kept missing or leaving events, making weak excuses to cover for me? My fear of being anything less than perfect haunted me. My mom expected me to behave and look perfect during my childhood visits with her, and I'd done my best to oblige. Now perfect was beyond my grasp. How, then, would I be worthy of Shelly's love? This wonderful, high-powered man who seemed to be out of my league when we first met was always reassuring me about how incredible I was. "You can sit next to a famous actor or the president of a large corporation and totally charm them," he would say. But it didn't register, all I could think of was that I needed to get a grip. I needed to get better. I couldn't keep having these episodes. I just couldn't.

As soon as we walked into our Beverly Hills condo, we flipped on the den television. Then we turned on the set in our bedroom as we peeled off our clothes, exchanging elegant black tie for comfy sweats, never taking our eyes off the show. With the removal of each restricting piece of clothing my pain subsided a little, and the tightness in my jaw relaxed a bit.

"I wish I'd set the VCR, " I said. "We missed the whole opening monologue, and I love Letterman." I glanced at the pool of taffeta and lace on the floor. It looked as deflated as I felt. I was losing control of the life I had dreamed of, the life I had achieved.

"I'll bring a tape home for you tomorrow. You get comfortable so we can enjoy the rest of the show," Shelly said.

It was so Shelly. The no-nonsense Shelly, who grew up in Brooklyn, the son of immigrant parents. By anyone's standards his family was poor, only he was never aware of that. What he knew was that he was surrounded by friends who played baseball, basketball, and stickball in the park every day and that his parents adored him. As president of television syndication in the black tower at Universal

Studios, Shelly never adopted the "entitled" attitude of so many Hollywood executives. He never demanded a certain table at a restaurant, he treated the guard at the studio gates with the same respect with which he treated his business colleagues, and he didn't need to wear diamond-encrusted gold watches or thousand-dollar shoes. Shelly was able to adapt to anything without feeling the least bit disappointed. He didn't pout. He didn't make me feel bad about anything.

I grew up in Los Angeles, the child of my divorced mom. Along with her twin sister, my Auntie Jo, they tried to raise me as best they could. I adored them both, but due to what they called "circumstances," I didn't get to live with them except on a weekend or a few days a month when they were off from their jobs as carhops at a hot local drive-in. Short skirts and majorette boots, combined with their good looks, equaled good tips, a nice apartment, and new cars. But there was no room for a young child in their always-changing work schedules. And so from the age of almost three until my mom remarried when I was nine, my mom paid for me to live in other people's homes, or "boarding out," as she called it. It wasn't under the foster-care system, simply people who took children into their homes to live for money. My mom always defended herself by saying this was the best she could do.

My dad was never around. He disappeared right before I started being boarded out. I didn't know him well enough to miss him. My mom and aunt never talked about him, it was almost as if he didn't exist.

As a child I equated love with disappointment and leaving, but an adult part of me always wanted to believe in love because of the television shows I watched, the movies I saw, and the books I read. They represented a world I didn't know as a child, but a world that I always wanted as an adult. I loved my mother despite the fact that she left me. Did she love me? I have asked that question of myself and even of my two half sisters, who were born much later when my mom remarried. The answer was unanimous: She loved as much as she could. My definition of love was jaded, unfulfilled, and distant. As an adult I didn't know how to trust and accept love until I met Shelly. Even with him, I held back, waiting for the other shoe to drop, waiting for him to leave. But being Shelly, he stayed.

As we made our way into our tiny den, Shelly stopped by the kitchen to pour tall glasses of iced mint tea. I sank into the comfy couch and rested my aching feet on the ottoman. Relief flooded my weary, inflamed body. My tears had stopped, but my eye makeup was a smudged reminder that we left the Oscars before they even started. Shelly sat next to me on the sofa and we clinked our glasses. "It's good to be home," he said, wiping away the mascara with his finger, as if he was the reason we were there. I still couldn't believe we'd left the pageantry of the live show to watch it on TV, but as I too felt the comfort and coolness of our home, as the medication started kicking in, and as I felt the love of a man who understood, I knew this was where I needed to be. Like millions of viewers all over the world, we sat in front of our television and were caught up in the excitement of the show.

The telephone startled us. Who calls during the Academy Awards? Most of our friends and family knew we would be at the show. Shelly could never let a phone go unanswered, and so he picked it up.

"Hey, how you doing? Yes, we decided not to go this year. Need a break." I knew by the tone of Shelly's voice that he had no idea who he was talking to.

"She's right here . . ." he said, handing me the phone.

"Steve, ah, Steve Hartman, what a surprise hearing from you. Aren't you working the show?" I asked him, mouthing to Shelly, "The reporter from CBS, the one I styled last month, remember? Dinner, you met him." He nodded.

"No, you couldn't have seen us, we're here, sitting in front of our TV," I lied. I tried to sound as convincing as I could, but he was as persistent then as he had been in his red-carpet interviews.

"Hey Steve, you must be working too hard, I'm sitting here in my sweats watching Meryl Streep at this very moment. Yes, we'll go shopping soon; I'll call you to set up a date. Glad the new clothes are working. Yeah, I got a call from the news director, and he likes the direction we're taking. Talk to you next week."

I hung up and looked over at Shelly. He didn't say a word. He understood why the cover-up was necessary. Before rheumatoid arthritis, lying was something I wouldn't consider doing. After rheumatoid arthritis, it became a necessity. I didn't feel guilty. Lies were the only way to keep this disease a secret, and there was no doubt in my mind that it must be kept a secret. One of the key components of my job was the use of makeup cover-ups, those flesh-colored concealers that hide flaws. For television I used cover-up on the makeover candidates, making them appear flawless. Now I used verbal cover-ups to hide my disease.

Shelly and I knew that in the worlds of fashion and entertainment in the early nineties people were not sympathetic about disease, especially one that was associated with disfigurement and aging. I was young, physically fit, madly in love, and at the pinnacle of my fashion career. How could I suffer from arthritis, a disease of old people with crippled hands and feet?

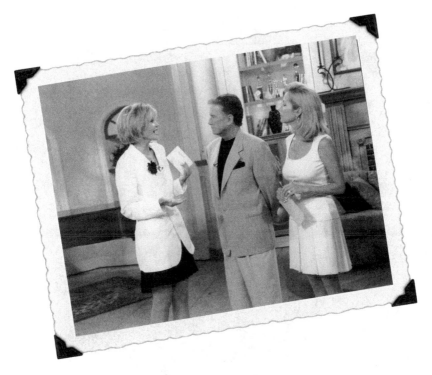

"Being on camera with Regis and Kathie Lee was such a positive experience. They always made me smile."

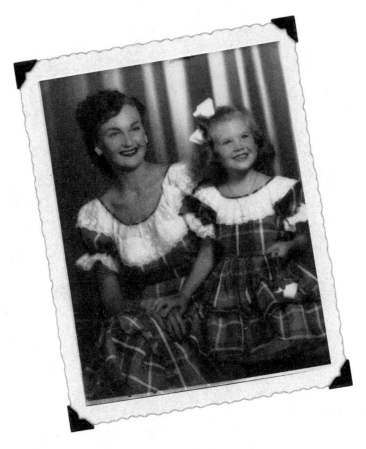

"I loved dressing up just like my mom. She was my fashion inspiration."

2

Sneakers to the Rescue

I was at the top of my game professionally, working on some of the most popular talk shows on television. I was happy in my personal life. I had been married for five months to my soul mate and best friend. My mother would have warned me in her "the glass is always empty" philosophy that it all seemed too good to be true. And as it turned out, it was.

I was working in New York on makeovers for Regis and Kathie Lee the day my first symptoms started. It seemed that out of nowhere my feet began throbbing. With each step on the busy sidewalks of the city I felt shooting pains bolt up through my feet toward my knees. My immediate thought was that I had overdone it on the treadmill. I can be a bit manic at times. A slice of cheesecake for dinner will drive me to an extra thirty minutes on the treadmill at an elevated level. I attribute it to the Jewish guilt I was learning from my new husband. And because I was well aware of the extra ten pounds the camera puts on, I had a tendency to add on those extra treadmill miles right before a television appearance. I guess you could say I was more than a bit manic.

Then it crossed my mind that my shoes were too narrow. I quickly dismissed that because they were the most incredible heels I owned. How could anything so beautiful be so painful? No, it had to be the treadmill. A good pair of sneakers would suffice through the next few days of schlepping to and from stores for styling around New York. Yes, sneakers, I would buy a pair right away.

The air had a crispness to it that let everyone know summer was over. Flying leaves floated gently to the sidewalks. Golden browns, mossy greens, and nearly pumpkin-orange leaves were highlighted against the blue sky. They crunched as I gingerly stepped on them with my beautiful but today painful black patent Jimmy Choos. Doormen from the hotels, busboys from the restaurants, and owners of small markets swept leaves into oversized trash bags to keep them from blowing inside as customers came and went. It was a hopeless job.

My job? To make over three women who had entered a contest on *Live with Regis and Kathie Lee*—three women who were beyond excited about the transition ahead of them. We selected them because of their potential for change. Often a good hardship story helped, but bottom line, the more I could visually change a makeover candidate, the higher the ratings. A good phone interview helped, but I had learned that there was very little television time for them to talk. It was all about the before-and-after photo. I also learned not to get too close to the candidates, a good lesson for all of television, where coworkers disappear faster than extras in a horror movie. I would have to do whatever was necessary to make changes, and I needed to keep my objectivity. Personally I liked pleasing people. Professionally I only had to please the cameras. The two were not even closely related.

I headed back to the Essex House Hotel, but not before stopping off at a corner shoe store. A new pair of cushioned sneakers hugged my swollen feet. My beautiful heels were tossed carelessly into one of the many shopping bags I carried. Each bag contained the components of the outfits I needed for the three makeover women I would dress at the studio in the pre-dawn hours the next morning. Earlier in the day my assistant had dropped off an equivalent number of packages at my hotel.

The doorman smiled when he saw me coming. "Good afternoon, Ms. Kunzelman . . . ah, sorry, I keep forgetting you're Mrs. Schwab now. Let me take those packages for you." He pried the tangled handles from the deep indentations they made on my hands. "There're some deliveries for you." Professionally I was still using my Kunzelman name, not wanting anyone to think I was trying to ride the Schwab coattails. Still, hearing the name outside the studios often took me by surprise.

"It's confusing, I'm Schwab in my personal life and Kunzelman on TV; you can call me either one. Will you run these up to my room?" I asked. I was overdue at the salon to check on the progress of my makeover's hair color.

"Of course, Madam" he answered, smiling at the generous tip I placed in his palm. Over the eight years I had worked in television I had learned that good tips equaled good service. I didn't have the luxury of time for locating lost packages or hailing my own cabs. I also had an understanding for anyone who worked in any business that depended on someone appreciating your talents.

My business was all freelance. I worked from job to job. Luckily I had a lot of work, but the fear always loomed when one job was over if there would be another. Childhood insecurities made it hard for me to believe that anything was permanent.

My first "boarded out" home was with my mom's friends Lorraine and Ray. They couldn't have children, so when my mom approached them about taking me in they were ecstatic. After only about six months, according to my mom, they became too attached to me. My mom, being young and insecure herself, felt threatened and moved me on to my "boarded out" home No. 2, Mama Dorothy's. There was no chance that Mama Dorothy would ever become too attached to anything but the monthly check my mom wrote.

Now I was on a regular, yet still freelance, schedule with Regis and Kathie Lee. I came to New York once a month and appeared on the show sometimes for one day, other times for a three-day series and about four times a year for a week of makeovers. For fashion segments I would stay in the city for three days: one to style, one on air, and the third to return merchandise and fly home. A week of makeovers kept me in the city for about seven or eight days. Fashion segments were a formula, but each makeover was like starting over. A new person, a new challenge, and a daunting time constraint. For each day of makeovers I had only twenty-four hours to do everything necessary before going on live national television. There was no room for error, and I needed all the help I could get.

The preparation for my work was not glamorous. Frantic and stressful, but never glamorous. The first day was putting it all together—clothes, hair, any necessary facial treatments like waxing, brow shaping or tinting, sometimes even dental work. The next morning on-air would be the payoff, and it had to be sensational.

My packages now safely at the hotel, I headed up 57th Street toward the salon. For anyone who hasn't walked up 57th Street, one of the busiest streets in the city, it is quite the experience. The wide sidewalks were shoulder-to-shoulder with people moving in both directions, somehow making it all work without too many major collisions. You could tell the New Yorkers because they weaved their fast-paced bodies in and out around the tourists. They crisscrossed the streets, taking advantage of the stoplights that would halt you in your tracks for what seemed like forever. You could spot the tourists because they were busy looking up at all the interesting buildings and the store windows not only on the street level, but on the second and third levels, making them quite dangerous to other tourists who were also looking up. Unlike in most cities, some of the most prominent stores, salons, and galleries were on the higher levels. The poor visitor who stopped to window-shop was quickly reprimanded for halting the flow of walkers.

I made my usual stop for an afternoon coffee-to-go. "Iced coffee, extra light, half decaf, half regular, with sweetener. To go," I ordered, searching for the mesh money bag in my oversized tote. Before I could get the money, the coffee was bagged and ready. It never ceased to amaze me how fast people could do everything in New York. Pity the poor tourist who needed to decide what he wanted to order when locals were lined up behind him. The coffee tasted delicious. Icy cold, but never weak and diluted in the summer and always boiling hot in the cold winter, none of those safe, lukewarm cups we got in Los Angeles. Butterscotch colored, just the way I liked it, and sweetened to perfection. I slowed my pace, just enough to enjoy my coffee without stopping foot traffic and savor each sip as I made my way back to the salon. I looked down at my aching feet. They bulged over the sides of my new sneakers and felt as if they were squished into one size too small. Had my size-nine feet grown to a size ten overnight? But enough about my feet. I had to keep my attention on what awaited me at the salon—what I knew from experience would be pandemonium.

The door of the prestigious Chanel-building elevator let me off at the third floor, home of the Frédéric Fekkai five-story salon. Chanel had recently bought the salon, but the talented staff and Frédéric remained in place. Every time I entered the salon the beauty of both the people and the interior took my breath away. Beautiful people working on beautiful people. Exquisite decor created what looked like a set out of a Hollywood movie. The motif was country French—expensive, tasteful country French.

My assistant, Bonnie, rushed into the elevator to greet me.

"We have problems," she whispered. I wasn't the least bit surprised. We always had problems getting artistic, creative hair-dressers and colorists to do what we wanted on makeover contestants who were sleep deprived from being put on a plane hours after being notified they had won a trip to New York. Most of them were, for the first time, visiting a city more populated than their entire home state. We'd spend the whole morning rushing from store to store to find the perfect TV outfit, nothing remotely close to anything they had ever seen, let alone worn. Add to all that the confusion of having their hair talked about as if it were not even attached to their heads. No wonder they so often had meltdowns. It was not unusual for a makeover to cry over hair that now lay on the floor in soft puddles of curls, or a new hair color that was unlike anything they had ever seen, let alone wore. Pair that with being overtired because of travel to New York, the excitement of the city, and the anticipation of being on live television the next morning and you have the ingredients for tears. Sometimes they are upset because of the physical change, but more often from the overwhelming, once-in-a-lifetime television experience.

As Bonnie led me over to the stylist's chair I saw the "problem" waiting for me, and as usual it was about hair color. Even with the best colorist in the business, making dramatic color changes for television was difficult. They had to work with hair they had never seen before, often overcolored by inexperienced people using home products. It was always a challenge.

"We must get life into this color," I demanded, brushing through dull brown hair that looked as if it had never seen the sun. "I want to lighten the base to a rich golden brown and then add highlights in two shades of creamy caramel." I looked deep into the eyes of the colorist, who was already thinking this would take six hours while knowing we only had two. Silently I pleaded with him not to say out loud that our contestant's hair was over-permed and that this would not be healthy.

When it came to television we cared only about what we would see on the screen. We were competing with all the other shows doing makeovers, so the stakes for the show and for me as a television talent were high. It was cutthroat. I knew what we did to our makeovers was selfish and sometimes damaging. No stylist in a working salon would have made as many changes in one day as we had to in order to satisfy the producers, the critical television cameras, and the TV audience. By then I knew the game and rationalized that my contestants were being treated like queens while being processed to the max for the greedy television cameras. After all, through that royal treatment, they'd come away with a wonderful new look that might even change their lives.

"Results, Christine, are ALL we care about. The sound of the audience as we reveal the before and after, the loud *Ahhh* reverberating into millions of homes around the country. Then we put them on the plane home," the executive producer had always said. Translated: "To hell with them, make drastic changes." In the early days of my career I balked and fought back until it became apparent that you did not fight back with an executive producer if you wanted to keep working. His stern, cold reply was always some variation of "We work in television," as if that were a higher calling, like healing the sick. So I adapted by being upbeat and positive with the makeovers. They were excited for the opportunity and as the producer said, "We're flying them to New York, putting them up at a good hotel, and picking up their expenses, not to mention the makeover, the free clothing, and the television exposure." I could see both sides, but most of all I loved my work and I needed to adapt, because the show was not going to adapt to me. The television industry often had little heart.

Running his fingers through the perm-damaged hair, the colorist played along. "Perfect, exactly what I was thinking. My darling, you will look like Christie Brinkley, you will be a goddess," he gushed as he caressed her hair. Before she could comment, the stylist moved in with his scissors and comb, and we continued our professional banter.

"What are your thoughts, Anthony?" I asked, as I leaned toward the woman's ear to whisper, "Anthony does Nicole Kidman AND Catherine Zeta-Jones . . . he is totally AMAZING."

"Oh Christine, this is an easy one, she has the features of Meg Ryan. I'm thinking we take it all off, a really short, spiky bob, one side tucked behind her ear, very saucy and sexy," he purred as he tucked a long straggly piece of hair behind one ear, only to reveal an overly large, forward bent, cauliflower ear. "Well, maybe we feather it around the face," he recovered quickly, folding the hair to a high-cheekbone length that covered the ear. "Yes, that's it, perfect, you will look FABULOUS darling, just fabulous."

Because it was always a battle for control in the salon, and I needed to keep the upper hand, I spoke up: "And just a few wispy bang pieces to float gently above her eyes."

"Perfect," Anthony said as he turned to face his assistant. "Philippe, will you take our beautiful makeover to start her color, we haven't a second to waste." Makeover No. 1 was whisked away. I found numbers easier than names, because there were so many makeovers and so little time. I never directly called them a number. I used enduring pet names—"sweetie," "doll," and "honey" worked just fine. No. 1 was savoring the sexy musk smell of the leave-in conditioner being massaged into her hair.

"How are our Makeovers No. 2 and No. 3?" I asked Bonnie, preparing myself for the complications that always arise when I have three makeovers to complete in one day. Bonnie pulled me to the side. We had learned that keeping the hairdressers happy was as hard as keeping the producers happy; egos are egos, they all were gigantic.

"You better check the color on No. 2," Bonnie said. "It's way too red. I tried to tell them, but they just blew me off. Her overly bleached blond hair has a lot of breakage. Fortunately she had her head back in the sink and couldn't see what washed down the drain. We've wrapped her head in a towel, waiting for you." I glanced over to one side of the salon and saw Makeover No. 3 in a brown silky smock with her client informational card tucked in the pocket, like a car needing to be serviced. At the time I wasn't aware that it was also like a patient in a hospital, dressed in one of their dreadful smocks with the medical chart clipped to the end of their bed.

"She's in shock with the color, thinks it looks black," Bonnie whispered.

"Let's see No. 3, the dye-back, first," I answered. A dye-back is a head of hair that is overbleached and usually a straw consistency, a head of hair that has simply lost all resemblance to hair. The solution is to put color back into the hair. The problem is that the overporous hair doesn't want to hold lighter colors, but it sucks up dark colors, making them appear darker than intended. Add to that a woman who is used to looking at herself with the palest of hair, and even a deeper blond color looks black to her in contrast. Experience had taught me that every dye-back thought her hair looked black. In this case, as I removed her tightly tucked turban towel, I saw it actually did.

"Ah," I murmured with what I hoped was a comforting voice, "the perfect base color for some soft tone on tone. "I ran my fingers through her mushy, spaghetti-textured hair. "Let's dry a small patch in the back and check, but it looks to me like we're right on target. Paris," I smiled my sweetest smile at the finicky hairdresser with the purple streaks in her hair, "I think our lovely lady deserves a steaming cappuccino."

Turning my full attention to the overtired, overwhelmed lady in the chair, I cooed, "Isn't this the most amazing salon? You know people come from all over the world to have their hair done here, for thousands of dollars. Between your hair and your outfit, you'll be a million-dollar baby tomorrow morning when you're standing in front of the cameras." I turned the chair away from the mirror so she could sip her cappuccino while we dried a piece of hair and figured out where to go from here. This would require a private conference. This would require some magic.

No. 2, the redhead, was indeed too bright. Given the hot lights and the cameras that would bear down on her in the morning, she risked looking like a dancer at a strip bar. "Let's give her a delicate brown glaze for shine," I said, which translated to, "Tone this sucker way down, we can't have clown hair on TV. Bonnie, I brought some cookies from the bakery, they're in a box by my tote, perfect with our coffees." I plopped myself down between the redhead and the dye-back, both to get off my still-aching feet and to keep the makeovers from talking to each other.

"What about manicures? We must have lovely nails for their debut. Bonnie, can you arrange for manicures while we put the finishing touches on their hair color?" I used my most positive tone, then I pulled Bonnie aside and whispered, "I've got to run to the store and pick up some Tylenol."

"But Christine, you can't leave now," Bonnie frantically pleaded.

"Bonnie, if I don't get something to ease this throbbing headache I'll go berserk. You can handle this. I'll be right back." I hated lying to Bonnie and leaving her to deal, but after all the running around the city, my feet hurt so badly that the pain was almost unbearable. It was either go around the corner to someplace where I could sit and slip my sneakers off and rub my aching feet for a few minutes or go crazy. I opted for the sneaker break.

Glancing at my watch, I realized Shelly must be wrapping up the day at his New York office and heading back to meet me at Cafe Luxembourg across town. I might be able to reach him in time to change our plans. I was just not up for going out to dinner, emotionally or physically.

"Shelly, let's have dinner at the hotel. I'm beat and it's going to be at least another hour before I can meet you. I've got to be at the studio by 5:00 in the morning, I hate to change our plans, but . . ."

"No problem, I'll call the Shaws and tell them we can't make it tonight and meet you back at the hotel. Don't rush, we can order up whenever you get back."

It still took me by surprise how nothing was a problem with Shelly. We'd somehow seamlessly combined our two hectic schedules. He usually planned his monthly business trips to New York to coincide with my television work or I planned my trips around his New York schedule. Regardless of how busy or tired we were, being together was more important. I could be researching a fashion shoot on my computer while Shelly caught up with *Variety* and *The Hollywood Reporter* and classical music played on the stereo. As long as we could spend time in the same room, we were happy. I felt adored.

> *Adored was not a word associated with my childhood. The move to Mama Dorothy's, as I look back on it now, was like taking someone out of a warm environment and dropping them off in the Antarctic. Mama Dorothy took in children, not to adore them, love them, or see that they flourished under her roof, but rather to make money to pay her bills. She fed us and kept us clean. I don't remember any laughter. I don't remember any warmth. She ruled her household with fear, of what I am not certain. All I do remember is living for each visit with my mom and my Auntie Jo and dreading each return to Mama Dorothy's. Her impatience and temper would fly, and for those of us living in her house, we never knew who would be the unlucky recipient. I do remember that I never wanted it to be me.*

Recently I was having a harder and harder time keeping up with Shelly's energy. It seemed like overnight I needed more rest, which even at forty-three was unheard of for me. Shelly could get by on four or five hours of sleep a night. Five minutes of downtime after a busy day, and he was ready for a business dinner. Lately I didn't feel like myself. Walking distance's that I never thought twice about before now seemed painfully long. I looked for places to sit where I would usually stand. The more I sat, the more I noticed others seeking out resting places. We looked at each other, almost as if knowing something was wrong. The secret club of people looking for a moment of relief in the form of a bench, a chair, a stool, or a leaning place. What I didn't know at the time was that fatigue was a symptom of rheumatoid arthritis. At the time I didn't even know what rheumatoid arthritis was.

Everything from grabbing coffee out to going through my mail now required a chair. Trying to keep up with Shelly's weight training in the gym caught up with me, too. I told myself next week, when we returned home, I'd take some downtime to make myself whole again. I tried to console myself that I was just tired, just pushing too hard, and putting in too many treadmill hours.

Deep down I worried. This felt like something more than just being tired.

3

Gulping Tylenol

OCTOBER 1990

New York was always exciting, but hotel living, when it's not a vacation but rather a working trip, can become claustrophobic. Rooms in New York are very expensive, small, and often dark if you are not facing the park or a wide street. We were lucky, we had good relationships with a few of the nice hotels, and because both Shelly and I were regulars, we were often upgraded to park views or larger rooms. But during busy travel seasons when hotels were sold out all over the city, we were lucky to get a room. So coming home to our light and airy condo one block east of Beverly Drive, right off Wilshire Boulevard, was always a treat. We were in the heart of the city while looking out large windows at trees filled with sunshine and the beautiful hills of Hollywood close by. Even the heaviest traffic in Beverly Hills seemed tame compared to the honking horns and jammed-up cars and taxis in New York. Beverly Drive was bustling at lunchtime with business people, but compared to the streets of New York it seemed empty.

I had decorated our condo in whites and beiges, with overstuffed, welcoming couches and chairs, the exact opposite of Mama Dorothy's dark and uninviting house. Everything at Mama Dorothy's was covered in plastic covers or runners to keep it clean and keep us—her boarders—from damaging her home. When I sat in shorts or a skirt on her couch my legs would stick to the plastic. Some of the plastic was old and cracked and scratched and pinched my skin. But we weren't encouraged to sit anywhere except at the cold chrome kitchen table or on the floor. "Crisscross applesauce," Mama Dorothy always said as she pushed us down on the floor and jerked our legs into the sitting position. But even the carpeted floor was covered in plastic runners.

When we returned home to our condo in Beverly Hills, after this last New York trip, things did not look as good to me because I was looking at them through tainted colored glasses.

On the third day home, I went to Century City shopping center to buy a birthday gift for a friend. The parking lot was underground, so I circled around trying to find the closest open space, but everything was filled. The only spot I could find was far from any escalator to the mall, and by this time even getting in and out of the car had become not only painful but also awkward. Trying to scoot forward in the seat took strength from my feet and knees that I didn't have. Until now I never noticed that car seats are slanted toward the back, so you fall into them. Getting dressed was agonizing, and walking caused excruciating pain with each step, beginning in my feet and quickly moving up my legs. I'd never thought about the number of steps from my car to any destination. Now I feared each one.

"Something's wrong with me," I had told my family doctor a day earlier. "I think I picked up a little flu bug from the airplane travel. My body aches all over, hurts when I move, and I'm excessively tired."

"Were you exposed to the flu?" he asked, stethoscope to my chest.

"I'm not sure, who knows what germs are flying around for the five hours on a plane to New York? I also overdid it on the treadmill and might have pulled a tendon or something in my feet. I can hardly walk in anything but sneakers. Maybe it's a combination of the treadmill and all the walking last week in New York." I tried a little too hard to convince him this was a sports injury—or was I trying to convince myself? "I had a foot massage in New York last week and it seemed to help. I even put shoe pads in my sneakers, but now I'm home, and whatever it is seems to be getting worse." I rattled on and on as he removed my shoes and looked at my swollen feet.

I jerked my foot back from his painful prodding and squeezing. "Hey, they're tender," I complained as I watched each toe turn from red to white as his thumb pressed into them.

"Your lungs sound fine, but there's definitely something going on with your joints, especially your feet. I'm going to refer you to an orthopedic surgeon for X-rays."

I remember being relieved. Orthopedic, right, now we're on track. Just as I thought, too much treadmill, a torn ligament for sure. A little physical therapy, and I'd be good as new.

I was calmer, thinking that this was definitely a sports injury. I tried to ignore the fact that the pain had become more intense. I circled round and round in the Pavilion's parking lot, my grocery list in my lap. Every close parking space was still taken. I couldn't consider walking any distance. I hung back, waiting for someone to leave so I could nab a space close to the door. Eventually someone pulled out only a few feet from the entrance. But I would need help just getting through the store. The shopping cart became a godsend. I found that if I leaned on it, I could take some pressure off my feet. I was getting more perplexed about how difficult it was to do everyday chores. Part of me believed I was just overdoing, but part of me feared it was more.

Two days later, the orthopedic doctor found nothing wrong with me and referred me to a rheumatologist, Dr. Terry Shack, whom I would see the next day. My fears spiked. I decided to focus on cooking dinner for Shelly rather than on my pain. It was one of our rare evenings at home, and we were both looking forward to it for different reasons. Shelly longed for a home-cooked meal and a baseball game on TV. For me it was a night I didn't have to get dressed up, make idle business chatter, and pound Tylenol to manage my pain.

By the time Shelly walked in the door at 7:30 the apartment smelled like Il Pastaio, one of our favorite Italian restaurants. It was a night of pasta with fresh tomato sauce, garlic bread, and a butter lettuce, mandarin orange, toasted almond, and avocado salad. I didn't have the energy to make a trip to the bakery for Shelly's favorite chocolate-chip babka for dessert so it was nonfat coffee yogurt from our freezer. I was fast asleep on the couch in the den, the Mets baseball game already in the fifth inning.

Leaning over to kiss me, Shelly whispered, "Hey, Sleeping Beauty, I smell delicious things from the kitchen—looks like you've been busy. I'm starving. I'll open a bottle of Chianti and get washed up. Why don't we eat in here so we can watch the playoff game?"

Blinking myself awake, I tried to focus on where I was, but the only thing I could focus on was my pulsating feet. Gingerly I stood up, holding on to the table next to the couch for balance. My God, what was going on in my body? I felt ninety instead of forty-three. Desperate for Tylenol, I shuffled to the bathroom, where Shelly washed his face and enthusiastically told me about his busy day—meetings here, deal signings there, and selling a big show into syndication, all part of a productive day's work for him.

"And what about you, what did you do today?" he asked, drying his face.

Washing down four Tylenols, I launched into my high-energy fabrications about all the things I'd accomplished when actually I didn't have a job lined up until the following week, and my fatigue had prevented me from making the necessary calls and e-mails to book anything.

"Worked the phones all morning, some solid gym time and then the market for tonight." I couldn't tell him I spent most of the day in and out of bed, trying to work up enough energy to do the grocery shopping and cooking for our small dinner. How could I counter a high-functioning day with a nonfunctioning one, especially when I had no explanation as to why I couldn't seem to get anything done? How could I explain to Shelly that getting in and out of my car was an effort? I loved to power walk the streets of Beverly Hills, absorbing each store window as a fashion research project. That was the Christine he knew and loved. Now I was a snail married to a racehorse. Today I had seen myself in the market's glass door as I laboriously made my way from the parking lot and the image stopped me in my tracks. Who was that hunched-over, waddling woman shuffling in her sneakers? It could not be me.

My mom was crazed about good posture, and because I was always tall for my age I had a tendency to slump. I'm surprised that there is not a permanent hand mark on my back between my shoulder blades where my mom always smacked her hand as she told me day after day as a teenager to stand up straight. There is hardly a time when I'm on the television set waiting for the red camera light to go on that I don't hear my mother's words in my head and quickly push my shoulders back and lift my head up by the imaginary string attached to the crown she always talked about. It was a good thing my mom was at home in San Diego now, most likely in front of her television watching some old movie, smoking and drinking strong black coffee, waiting for her beloved cocktail hour so she could start pouring wine. Even sitting in her oversized reclining TV chair, I knew her posture was perfect.

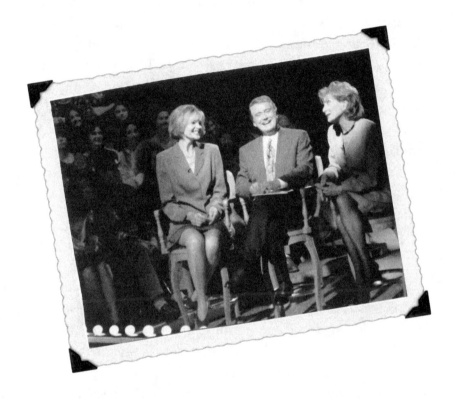

It was a thrill working with two television icons, Barbara Walters and Regis Philbin.

4

No Time for Derailment

I tried to imagine that Shelly and I were going to Westwood for dinner and a movie like we usually did. Today, instead of making a right turn into the theater parking lot, we made a left turn into the UCLA Medical Center, where my world would soon fall apart. When Shelly heard the message on our answering machine confirming my appointment at UCLA, he canceled his day. He was determined to get to the bottom of what was bothering me.

"UCLA. Great, Christine, they'll figure it all out and you'll be like new," he said. How could I be like new when I felt so old? I had been on strong anti-inflammatories for three months now from my first rheumatologist, Dr. Shack, and instead of feeling relief I was getting worse. Dr. Shack couldn't come up with a diagnosis. My blood work was not showing anything definitive. When he did the physical test of squeezing and moving the joints in my feet there was pain, but pain from exactly what was not defined. Now I had both the pain in my body and an upset stomach from the medications. Dr. Shack, frustrated at his inability to confirm what was wrong with me and find medications that would help, recommended I see a cutting-edge doctor at UCLA. Today was my appointment day.

Westwood Village sits at the entrance to the UCLA campus. It's a charming college town filled with casual restaurants, trendy stores, and large movie theaters whose marquees sparkled at night. This morning we were bypassing the charming village and heading straight onto the campus for my first appointment with Dr. Ken Kalunian. The sidewalks were clogged with rushing students and doctors dressed in everything from colorful scrubs to crisp white monogrammed jackets. Community service buses pulled up to the curbs, dropping off patients with canes, walkers, and wheelchairs. Limo drivers assisted their well-dressed clients out of cars, many with grave faces, clutching large X-ray envelopes that held the stories of their new diseased lives. There were few things that could equalize the poor and the rich, the educated and noneducated as quickly as the hospital entryway. Here we all had one thing in common: We were suffering and desperate for help.

UCLA Medical Center was where people came for the answers they couldn't get anywhere else. My mind did a quick flashback to the parking lot at ABC Studios, where I recently carried bags of accessories for a style segment on their morning show. As I walked toward Studio 2, I passed actors dressed in doctor costumes walking into Studio 4, where they taped General Hospital. Handsome and beautiful faces made up to perfection, scrubs starched and pressed. Actors playing doctors and patients on a television show. Today, at UCLA, the stark contrast between my television fantasy world and my medical world was overwhelming.

Here I stood at the entrance of the medical building, wishing I was at the ABC studios, where it was all make-believe. Instead I was a real patient making my way to the department of internal medicine and a third-floor waiting room filled to capacity with people who looked disheveled, stressed, and ill with very real diseases.

"I need to copy your insurance card, Mrs. Schwab," the nurse behind the counter called out to me.

"You sit, I'll do it," Shelly said, jumping up before I could even move my aching body to the front of the chair.

I turned the pages of my December issue of *Vogue* without knowing what I was reading. My anxious stomach competed with my tender feet and knees for attention—both were killing me.

Shelly read to me, trying to add some levity, as he folded his newspaper in neat, small sections in that cramped New York subway style of reading papers in public places.

"Actress Jennifer Aniston, who portrays Rachel on the TV show *Friends,* inspires a craze for a longer version of the shag haircut. Women across the country are demanding that their hairstylists give them the 'Rachel' or *'Friends'* cut, a face-framing, multilayered look."

After what seemed like an entire morning, a harried nurse escorted us into a small examining room. Decor was not important at UCLA; the room had all the charm of a free clinic in an otherwise boarded-up row of stores. The grayish green patient room was crammed with peeling metal furniture. The examination table was covered in white paper; a fold-down desk was stacked high with blank prescription pads. A rolling tray and stool stood ready for the doctor, both lined up perfectly with all the dents and scratches along the walls. With barely room to walk, we quickly found seats, Shelly in a stack chair while I sat on the exam table. A young intern came in to take my information. He neither looked at me nor talked to me. He talked at me with a list of routine health questions.

"Any major illnesses?"

"No."

"Surgeries?"

"Do eye lifts count?"

"Have you ever been hospitalized?"

"Only twenty-three years ago when my son was born."

"Allergies?"

"Codeine."

He scribbled my answers. I was a new chart to be filled out. No weight, height, or eye color. Little did I think the chart would soon be overflowing with symptoms.

After another hour the doctor entered. "Hi, I'm Dr. Ken Kalunian. I see by your chart that you have some pain going on in your feet and knees."

"Yes, I think I pulled or strained something from overdoing it on the treadmill, but they . . ."

My husband interjected, "Actually, the orthopedist ruled out any type of injury. Our family doctor and the rheumatologist weren't able to come to any conclusions, so we were referred to you." Shelly knew I was still holding on to the hope that this was a sports injury, a hope that was no longer realistic in his logical mind. I remained quiet. Normally I would have asserted myself and my opinions. This passivity wasn't like me. Had I pounded my assertive self into the treadmill along with my damaged feet?

Dr. Kalunian continued, "Looking over your X-rays, there's no indication of any type of injury. I'd like to do some blood tests, but first let's look at your feet and knees." I slipped off my sneakers and rolled my jeans above the knees. "Ouch, that hurts," I complained as the doctor squeezed my toes, which looked like they were filled with a watery gel, one at a time. His squeezes made those of the previous doctors seem gentle, or was it that my pain had increased, making me so much more sensitive?

"Definitely some inflammation; let's take your blood. We'll get the results today, so if you don't mind waiting a bit, once we have the information we can talk," he said, walking out of the room, seemingly anxious to get on to another patient. The nurse came in and took six vials of blood.

And we waited.

There was nothing of interest to look at in the room. There was nothing to talk about that was more important than what we were doing right then, and yet I couldn't talk about it. The fear of loss lingered in the claustrophobic air as I sat on the cold, paper-covered exam table. This was not my world. My world was healthy, beautiful, and stylish. My world, especially on television, made no allowances for any illness beyond a cold. What was I doing here, in this place, with all these sick people?

"I think we finally found the right place, Christine," my husband said in his most positive voice. I could hear the smile in his words and yet I couldn't smile.

"How do we know it's the right place? They've done exactly what the other rheumatologist did, only it's taking about three times longer."

I went back to turning the pages of *Vogue,* ending the conversation. I had nothing positive, informative, or interesting to say. I hurt. My feet throbbed. My knees screamed every time I moved them. My entire body seemed to be breaking down. I was exhausted and depressed. Instead of working on an exciting fashion segment for television, I was in an anonymous faded cotton smock at UCLA, a gigantic, bustling building full of sick people. Very sick people.

"Okay," Dr. Kalunian began as he opened the door and took a seat on the small swivel stool, "Based on your blood test today there is no definitive indication of disease."

My body heaved a sigh of relief. My joints ached.

"However, from my examination of your joints I feel confident that you have an early and mild case of rheumatoid arthritis. Because it's at such an early stage nothing is showing up in your blood yet."

ARTHRITIS.

Pictures of crippled people in wheelchairs at the television arthritis telethons flashed before my eyes.

ARTHRITIS.

Wasn't that a disease for old people? I was only forty-three. This could not be happening.

I opened my mouth to speak, but all that came out were frustrated, disbelieving, muffled sobs. My mind filled with visions of my mother, watching the arthritis telethon, her cigarette dangling between her lips as she said, "Look at those crippled people. I'd rather be dead, yes, just shoot me if I ever end up like that."

This young, self-assured, cocky doctor seemed happy to have found a niche to put me in. A diagnosis to fill my chart. Why did he have a smile plastered on his face?

"Well, this is certainly good news," my husband said, sounding relieved, he picked at the lint on my cotton gown, placing it in a neat ball that he rolled tightly in his palm. Control, my husband thought he was gaining control.

GOOD NEWS. Was he kidding? What was good about this?

"Actually, it is. I was concerned we had a case of lupus, which is a far more serious disease," Dr. Kalunian turned and talked directly to Shelly. I guess it was easier; he didn't have to deal with the terrified expression on my face. The only positive thing I could think of was how glad I was that I wasn't on television getting this diagnosis where I'd been trained to be ready for everything and hide any negative emotions, but this overwhelming information was way too much to hide.

"What exactly is rheumatoid arthritis?" my take-charge, let's-get-this-fixed husband asked.

I remember the doctor shifting into his professional training mode, sitting up taller, buttoning the top button of his lab coat, moving to eye contact with Shelly, pen poised in his right hand as he explained, "Most people think anything with the word arthritis in it is all one disease, but it's not. The most common disease is osteoarthritis, a wearing out of the joints that people acquire as they age. Rheumatoid arthritis, what Christine has, is an immune system disease, a type of arthritis that causes pain and swelling in many joints. The cause isn't known, but what is known is that both genetics and triggers from the environment seem to play big roles. You need to have a certain genetic pattern to be susceptible to the disease, but not all people with those patterns get the disease. It seems that you need a trigger from the environment to cause the genes to turn on and make antibodies that cause a patient to get symptoms. Basically the body attacks itself. Once you get symptoms, it's rare for it to go away on its own, and drugs are needed to decrease the symptoms."

Shelly absorbed it all, fascinated, relieved, and ready to tackle the problem as he did everything, straight on in his bulldog manner.

"Quite simply, the body attacks itself, eating at and destroying the joints," the doctor said as if he were telling us that I had the flu and with lots of liquids, it would go away in a week or ten days.

I observed the two of them engaged in their medical talk. It felt as if I was floating above the room and watching strangers talk about someone else. This couldn't be my life they were referring to. My life was finally on track. I had given birth to a son, survived a divorce, helped my son get started at USC, moved my career forward, and met and married my soul mate. I couldn't derail, not now, not when I finally had all the pieces in perfect place. Not when I was living the dreams that kept me hopeful through a painful childhood. My two sisters liked to call me Sparkle Plenty—because they said I always tried to put a positive spin on life, and I did, but not this day. This day I couldn't even begin to sparkle. Watching as Shelly listened intently to the doctor, I grabbed both sides of my head to stop the pounding. For the first time in a while, something hurt more than my feet.

"We're going to stop the anti-inflammatory Voltaren Christine's been taking and replace it with Naprosyn, which should be easier on the stomach. I'm also adding a low dosage of Sulfasalazine, which will also help reduce the inflammation and slow the disease's progress. I'll increase the drug as needed and prescribe some physical therapy at Cedars-Sinai. There are no apparent foot erosions, so our goal is to prevent any damage in the future. We'll keep a close eye on Christine," he continued, writing out a prescription and handing it to Shelly. "I want to see her back here in two weeks for more blood work. In the meantime if there's any questions or concerns please give me a call," and he handed the prescription and a couple of brochures with old, crippled people on the covers to Shelly, shook his hand, nodded at me and walked out of the room.

"Christine, Christine, why are you so sad? This is a good diagnosis. This isn't fatal. Now that we know what it is you can start to get better." Moving over to the examining table to hold my quivering body, Shelly tried to calm me down, but there was no calming. As he rubbed my back with one hand I saw the brochures in his other hand. They were hardly the *Vanity Fair* Hollywood covers. Instead of beautiful celebrities, they were filled with older people with crippled hands and feet. How could I be put in the same group with these victims of rheumatoid arthritis? How would I ever hold on to my life, my career, and my new vibrant and sexy husband? Right then, in that grayish-green cubicle of a room, in my husband's arms, I felt this wonderful life slip away, and I didn't know how to even begin to stop it. I was once again that small, scared, young child who watched her mother load the suitcases into the car for the third move to another "boarded-out" home.

"You'll love this new home, Chrissie. Margie and Bill have two kids around your age, plus other young boarders. It'll be a real family, you'll see, don't cry, you'll like it," my mother said, turning up the volume of the car radio to muffle the sound of my sobs.

But I didn't like it at Margie and Bill's. I didn't like their kids, and they didn't like me and yet I lived there for more than three years, until even my mom knew she would have to do something different. "Boarding-out" was simply not working. I had never had control of my childhood, and I now understand that most kids don't have control, but most kids live with their parents, or even one parent. But my mom always felt in control. I was in a safe, clean home, my dad was no longer around, and she was able to do her work and have her life. What I didn't recognize on her face that day she told me about my new boarded-out home was her awareness that she was also losing control. I was becoming so unhappy that in the future something would have to be changed. Maybe the turning up of the radio was not just to block out my sobs, but to cover up the pounding of her heart? Did she have any solutions? At the time I didn't have any idea the anxiety this was causing her, and she was trying to deny the anxiety it was causing me. Denial was becoming less and less of a solution.

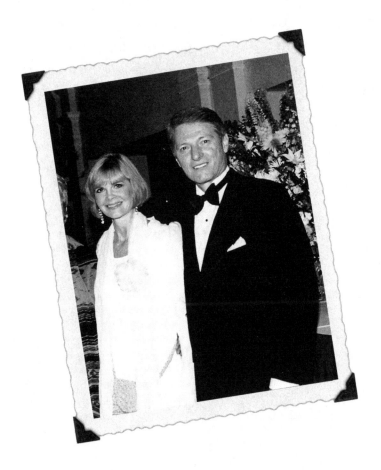

Perks of Hollywood include glamorous events like the Oscars, The Emmys, The Golden Globes, and the National Association of Television Program Executives.

5

Rockin' to the Pointer Sisters

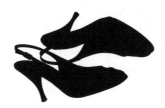

JANUARY 1991

I used all of my patience to lie on the padded table while my mind worked in overdrive thinking about all the things I needed to be doing at home. Having my hands and feet massaged and covered with warm paraffin wax, then stuffed inside heated gloves, was not one of those tasks. If I was in a salon selecting a polish color it would be lovely, but this physical-therapy treatment was supposed to help my fingers and hands from aching. The throbbing of my feet had now moved up from my knees to my wrists and hands. I squirmed on the hard table, smelled the camphor mixed with sweating bodies that filled the physical therapy room, stared at glaring, blinking fluorescents on the cracked ceiling, and listened to the chatter of the therapists as they worked with their patients at Cedars-Sinai Medical Center. I drifted off, dreaming of the familiar, safe little prairie house from my favorite childhood book where I was running and jumping, chasing my dog Sam, trying to catch him as he slipped through my big greasy, heated mittens.

The therapist goal today was to help me feel better for the upcoming NATPE (National Association of Television Programming Executives) convention in New Orleans, which was just six days away. I doubted that paraffin and massage would be the magical antidote, but hey, with pain I'd found that anyone would try anything, including me. I had bought a copper bracelet that was supposed to ease my hand pain, but all it did was bruise my wrist when I would bang into something. I had tried an amethyst ring that was supposed to strengthen my immune system, but the stone was large and it brought attention to my red, swollen fingers. My favorite ethereal purchase was a stone etched with the word "believe," because it made me think that if I believed I would be well, I would. Some days it worked better than others.

NATPE was the biggest professional convention of the year for Shelly. Being there for my husband was a social obligation, but the access to high-powered people was also good for my career. Shelly's schedule would be nonstop, morning to night, and most days I had to myself. I liked to walk the halls of the convention. I passed everybody in the business. Instead of trying to get through assistants and busy calendars on the phone, I could be in direct contact with the major players in those halls, making it easy to give a little PR-type pitch about what I was working on that might fit into something they had in progress. It was a major perk to be able to attend as the wife of Shelly Schwab. The four evenings would each be filled with mandatory business dinners and parties, and I was expected to attend.

That first day of diagnosis at UCLA was the worst day for me, because I was blindsided by the words "rheumatoid arthritis." I'm not sure if I borrowed my survival tool of denial from my childhood that day or not, but I was so positive—or at least I had convinced myself that I had a sports injury. Health had never been an issue for me. My career was based on promoting the image of a healthy, active, stylish woman. And still, even after the diagnosis, I hung on to the denial. I couldn't read any books on arthritis because they were so depressing. The so-called bible, *The Arthritis Cure,* sent me over the edge of depression. This wasn't me. I wouldn't, couldn't, allow it to be me. I would never let rheumatoid arthritis define who I was. I might have it, but it wasn't going to define me.

Luckily my follow-up meetings with Dr. Kalunian had improved. He talked to me now, because Shelly was at work. I had stopped crying, at least in front of the doctor. The shower, the car, and waiting rooms were another matter. I wouldn't admit I accepted this disease, but I at least came for my appointments. We were trying a new, stronger combination of drugs to take down the inflammation in my joints. It seemed to be the key to keep the swelling at a minimum, but the drugs were strong and played havoc with my stomach, making me queasy most of the time. Crackers replaced my favorite Oreo cookies as the staple in my purse. I feared I was becoming one of those little old women taking saltines from restaurants.

I was growing to like my doctor. We were getting to know each other. He understood my busy, demanding lifestyle. "Seeing you and Shelly together and hearing your schedules, I see the pressures on you to keep your life as normal as possible," Dr. Kalunian said, once again squeezing my joints to test for inflammation.

"And keep this disease under wraps," I added. "I have no doubt it would hurt my career and actually, I don't know how I could handle people knowing. I'm having a hard time dealing with it, let alone dealing with everyone else." I didn't mince words when I told him I must feel good and look good, and he seemed to feel he could make that happen. And because he already worked with a celebrity clientele, he knew he would have to keep all our efforts secret as he became my partner in hiding.

Me? I wasn't convinced. Visions of wheelchairs haunted my dreams. Of course the phone conversation with my mom the previous week didn't help.

"Mom, they finally figured out what's causing my pain. I have rheumatoid arthritis," and then I quickly went into my

"Sparkle Plenty" sales pitch. "But my doctor feels he's catching it early and will be able to keep it under control."

"Oh my God, Chrissie, arthritis? Are you sure? Half your father's family ended up in wheelchairs. You're too young to be crippled." Wow. A sentiment right out of Hallmark. There was no concealing the horror, even disgust, in her voice. She was the anti–Tony Robbins. "Sorry, Mom, I've got a call coming in that I have to take," I said to shut out her negativity. Another necessary lie. Once off the phone I knew she was right, at least about my dad's family.

I reflected back on my dad, a self-made and somewhat destroyed man. With no support from his family he went to college and got a bachelor's degree in engineering. He became successful with seven water-saving patents in his name, traveling the world teaching water conservation. He came back into my life when I was nine and living with my mom and new stepdad. He was a stranger I didn't know, a dad I never knew how to love because he never knew how to love me and yet we forged an odd, distant relationship, unlike any father and daughter I have ever known. Being his only child, I was the one who was there at the end of his life, and along with the hospice nurses kept him comfortable and, per his wishes, out of the hospital. Now I had arthritis just like my dad. In my hands and feet, just like my dad. Only unlike my dad, I was being proactive. My dad had chosen to ignore his disease. I refused to end up in a wheelchair as my mother predicted. I may have inherited some of my dad's denial, and some of his arthritis, but I was determined not to be like my father.

I lived for climbing into bed and stretching out. It was about the only place where I could relax. My husband lived for getting into bed to play. He had the sexual appetite of a twenty-year-old. As he was lighting candles and putting on music, I'd be aching all over. The mere thought of sex hurt my joints, but the thought of him filled me with lust. How could I abruptly change the great sex life we'd had to this point? I couldn't. This was a man who loved sex, and this was a man I loved. I kept my aches to myself, and we continued the life we had, or at least he thought we did. For me, the beginning and after of sex was painful, but the middle? I was lost in delicious passion. Relaxed and satisfied, he spooned next to me, already half asleep. I sneaked out of bed to take a pain pill, the euphoria of sex worn off and the reality of my tender joints returned. Soon I joined him in a sweet, chemically enhanced slumber, my new favorite part of the day.

In the morning it started all over again, the slow awakening of my body and my pain. It was as though when I started to stretch, I'd awaken the army inside me that quickly marched from feet to shoulders, raking fingernails across my nerve endings, irritating them to the point of throbbing pain. Every time I moved, the pain shot through a joint. I was aware of how many joints I had in my body, joints I never thought of before, now complaining when I activated them. To do something so basic as bending to pick up a piece of paper on the floor stressed my shoulders, elbows, wrists, fingers, hips, knees, and ankles. Each joint grumbled as I engaged it for such an everyday task.

By my first cup of coffee, my pain was at full throttle, and I wondered how I would get through the day. My days now consisted of very little. My only goal was to make it through the minimal amount of work I needed to do for my career and the business dinners and events I had to attend for Shelly's career. I canceled every appointment I could without causing suspicion. I was getting good at it. Some days I could even convince myself that I was normal, healthy, all the things I now pretended to be. My media contacts weren't suspicious. A quick excuse and then I would make it all about them: "I saw that special you produced. You are amazing." And "You're going to be running that network soon" always did the trick, putting the focus on them and taking it off me. "The camera caught you on the set yesterday as I was watching TV, and you looked incredible, what's your secret?" was another good deterrent. And they never thought to ask the second question about why I wasn't available or was rescheduling. I was still working, some weeks more than others. The only difference? My health now dictated how successful I could continue to be.

My latest excuse to friends went like this:

"I'm jammed with this *Entertainment Tonight* project about celebs getting ready for the Academy Awards. It's going to go on for weeks, and there's tons more to research. *ET* is demanding but it's *ET,* they get to be." And because it was a hot show that I had worked on special assignments for before, no one questioned my cancellations of breakfasts and luncheons. Much of my calendar was covered with Wite-Out, making way for my new appointments with pain.

Some days, my entire day would consist of a trip to UCLA for labs. It should have been easy, but it took hours of parking, sitting in the waiting room, taking labs, waiting for results, meeting with Dr. Kalunian for an update, adjustments in medicines and then home to rest up for the evening. At home, it took me twice as long to get myself ready for a night out because everything now exhausted me. Even blowing my hair dry was a chore. I was sure my hair dryer had gained weight; surely it couldn't have been this heavy before. The more active my disease, the more time and effort I spent dressing, styling my hair, and applying my makeup. Percocet took the edge off my pain but put me in a fog that made applying a straight line of eyeliner almost impossible. Ozzy Osbourne didn't have this much trouble putting on makeup. I used a damp Q-tip to adopt the smudged look, or as I started naming it for evening, "smoky eyes." For someone who had taught television viewers the "ten minute out the door in style morning routine" I was now the "two hour, barely out the door" fatigued example.

Appearance was the only thing that gave me the feeling of some control over my life. As I checked my clothes in the mirrored closet doors, my chocolate-brown evening suit looked chic. The three rhinestone pins I placed on the collar sparkled into my face. The brown fishnet nylons felt sexy and took the focus off my low-heeled, sensible, comfortable shoes. Sensible was not a word usually found in my fashionable vocabulary. My magnifying makeup mirror reflected a healthy face made-up with a touch of shimmer for evening. It surprised me that I looked so normal.

This night we were going to the Beverly Hilton for a charity black tie event honoring Sherry Lansing, the president of Paramount Studios. An hour of cocktails in the lounge area used to be an appointment for stimulating conversation with media moguls. Now I regarded it as an hour of standing on my aching feet, then painfully maneuvering my way through the crowds to a table occupied by the top executives at Shelly's company, Universal Studios. At least there I could sit, but that in itself created a problem when it was time to stand for an ovation. I pretended to do an outfit adjustment while getting my stiff feet and knees to work properly. I was getting good at hiding my disease. Often I'd whisper something in Shelly's ear as I stood, just enough time to stall and get my circulation moving.

"What's with the secrets?" Shelly asked, trying to hear my whispers in the noisy room. I'd just give him a little kiss and smile. Secrets were now my way of coping.

The evenings usually ended by ten o'clock. These were busy people who had early morning meetings and short attention spans. They were savvy people who went to many events during the week with the stipulation that they could be home at a decent hour. The challenge came in getting our car. Rude as it seemed, almost half the guests started heading for the exits during the last speech. Often we were part of that rude crowd. I moved so slowly that if Shelly didn't run ahead we would end up at the back of the valet line. How I felt determined how long our exit would take. The key was to walk and act as normal as possible. My RA had not made any physical changes in my appearance. No one outside my immediate family knew, and I intended to keep it that way. Really, in show business nobody cared about what was going on in other people's lives unless it could somehow translate to something that would benefit them. A new show, an upcoming party of the somebodies, or a hot new agent in town looking for clients could translate to potential work; those were topics that make people listen. Disease was certainly not.

Later that week we boarded Universal's private Gulfstream jet for New Orleans. It was usually empty, but on this particular day every seat was filled with presidents of the different divisions and their spouses.

"Best lox and bagels, where do they get this food?" Shelly asked one of his colleagues, who was also munching a bagel.

"They gather everyone's orders and send runners out to the best restaurants in the city. I think this is from Wasserman's favorite deli, Nate'n, Al in Beverly Hills," the coworker said.

"Taste this herring," Shelly handed me a fork filled with white- and silver-looking slime.

"No thanks, I'm fine with my crackers and cheese." The thought of adding herring to my already upset stomach was inconceivable.

The oversized leather airplane chairs were comfy and made the cross-country trip pleasurable. The open space made it easier to get up and walk. When we arrived at the small airport, black town cars were lined up, trunks opened and waiting for their important passengers. Such a spoiled, easy way to travel. These executives worked long and hard, but their perks were glamorous and indulgent. The company wanted them to concentrate only on business.

The Windsor Court Hotel in New Orleans was exquisite. The "conversation pit" in the center of the lobby was already filled with the who's who of television: Brandon Tartikoff, the head of the NBC Network, looking for new shows to buy.

Phil Donahue working to secure more outlets for his show, and Suzanne Somers pitching her pilot. Everyone drinking and promoting. Business had begun. Shelly stopped to visit while I went to the room to unpack for the King World party at the Superdome. King World always threw the party of the convention, sparing no expense for top-notch bands and extravagant decor. Tonight the Pointer Sisters were performing. Everyone would be there as the group rocked the football stadium, and the dance floor would be jammed. I packed my most comfortable shoes with padded inserts, and the doctor had given me permission to take an additional half a Percocet for pain if necessary. I wanted to be part of the party, too, but the question was, would I be able to? My joints seemed a little better from my increased drug regimen, but my stomach was churning.

"Hey, we better hustle, sweetie," Shelly asked, rushing into the suite two hours later, finding me dressed in my robe and lying on the bed, the heavy blackout drapes closed against the bright setting sun.

"You're not even dressed. Are you okay?"

"No, I'm not doing so well. My stomach's upset. I called Dr. Kalunian, and he said to call the hotel doctor. Something about ruling out internal bleeding from my medications," I answered, grabbing my stomach as it went into spasm from trying to reach for the glass of water by my bed.

"So when's the doctor coming?" Shelly asked, handing me the water. Even scooting up in bed for a sip was excruciating.

"I didn't call. I can't call a hotel doctor with everyone in this hotel being in the business."

"Christine, we're calling the doctor. This is crazy and could be serious," Shelly said, running his fingers through my tangled hair. "Yes, we need to get the hotel doctor to room 711 as soon as possible. My wife is having stomach pain, and her doctor at UCLA wants her checked out." Shelly spoke in his no-nonsense business voice. He could get anybody to do anything.

"They'll have someone here in twenty minutes. Can I get you anything?" he asked, laying out his outfit for the evening. "Why don't you get ready, so we can leave as soon as the doctor gives you the okay," Shelly glanced at me, trying to figure out why I looked so good when I complained of feeling so bad.

"I can't go, Shelly."

"But you've been looking forward to this party for weeks," he said, obviously thinking of the pre-RA Christine who wouldn't miss a party for anything. Anything. "The doc will give you something to settle your stomach, and you'll be good as new," Shelly said in his optimistic tone, as he changed his shoes.

"I don't think so. You need to go without me." Actually I wanted to be by myself, I didn't even feel like talking. Usually I could rally enough spirit to put on the smiling Sparkle Plenty face my family had come to count on. But not tonight. Tonight I couldn't even pretend.

"No, it's out of the question, I'll stay with you," Shelly said.

"No, you should go. This is a business trip."

Shelly was in his business mode—define the problem and solve it. I was in my pain mode; all I needed was empathy. I wanted to be alone in the dark, quiet room. I didn't even want to see the doctor. How was I going to get this disease under control when the medications seemed to be as harsh as the pain? I felt as if the insides of my body were taken over in some sort of revenge. Rheumatoid arthritis was eating at my joints and attacking my stomach in a mysterious and circuitous way. My orange plastic pill jars sat clustered together in the hotel bathroom, their names a blur, waiting to help me, hurt me, or blur the pain. I was beginning to think even the doctors didn't know which direction to take.

"Ohhh, that hurts," I complained as the doctor pressed on my queasy stomach.

"There doesn't seem to be internal bleeding, but I think you better stop taking your medications until you get back home and can see your doctor."

"But how can I function?" I asked, knowing that without any medications my joints would flare even more.

"The medications will stay in your body for a few days. Do you have anything for the pain?"

"Percocet."

"That should get you through. Keep your stomach coated with Maalox," the doctor said, packing up his little black bag. As he was leaving, he told Shelly, "She'll be fine. This is not unusual for patients on high dosages of anti-inflammatories."

The two of us alone again, I told Shelly, "Go, please, go to your party."

"Why don't you try to come just for a short time, make an appearance, and then we'll leave early?"

I understood how important it was to Shelly, how in his own way he was in as much denial as I was. I encouraged this denial by keeping some symptoms from him. Against all common sense, I decided to go. I couldn't bear for people to look at me as if I were sick, especially the man I loved. I gulped down Maalox and dressed. But the limo ride to the stadium was reality and way too much movement.

"Please, stop the car, I'm sick," I yelled to the driver, realizing I didn't have much time. And there on the side of the road, in my glamorous Calvin Klein outfit and black patent flat dancing shoes, I lost what little lunch of crackers and cheese I ate on the plane.

"Back to the hotel," my husband said to the driver as I climbed back into the car, embarrassed, humiliated, and slightly green. My stomach was rocking, but it wasn't to the Pointer Sisters.

I spent the rest of the convention in my room at the Windsor Court, eating boiled white rice and dry wheat toast. It was as bland as I felt. I watched the in-house convention news and tried to read. I realized I had turned fifty pages without absorbing a thing as I unconsciously tried to figure out this new life. The few people who noticed I was not around at the convention activities were satisfied with Shelly's brief "She's on deadline for *ET*" explanation. Amazing, the power of the words *"Entertainment Tonight."* I saved all my energy to greet Shelly at the hotel when he came home late from a day on the convention floor and a business dinner, exhausted and exhilarated, ready to tell me of his productive day. This role-playing on my part made me feel like I had at least some control of my life. My generation was the *Donna Reed, I Love Lucy,* and *Father Knows Best* happy housewife face. Problems were meant to be swept under the carpet. And sweep them I did. All safely tucked under the carpet of the Windsor Court Hotel. By the time I left New Orleans and headed home to get ready for my upcoming trip to New York, I gave off the impression of being the picture of health. In reality I was fighting for relief from a disease that was fighting for control. I often felt that the only reason I was able to survive was because of my ability to create a fantasy world. The same fantasy world that I used every time my mom took me back to my "boarded-out home." Without my ability to pretend, I doubt if I could have survived her constant leavings.

> *"Chrissie, promise me you won't cry when I take you back to Margie and Bill's today. I hate to think of you being so sad all week," my mom said as she picked up all my toys and put them back in the closet, returning her beautiful apartment to its childless, pristine state. I looked around. Not one sign of me was left. Erased. All packed away, like my little Cinderella suitcase standing ready by the front door. Our mother-daughter weekend was over until the next time.*

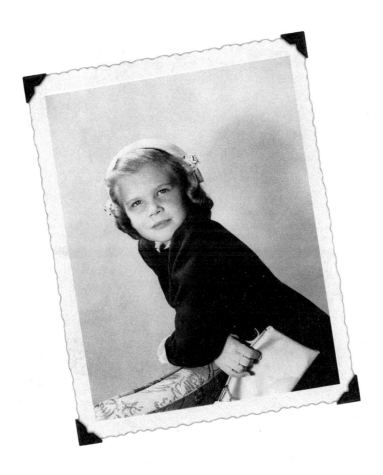

Does the camera capture my sadness or am I the only one who sees it?

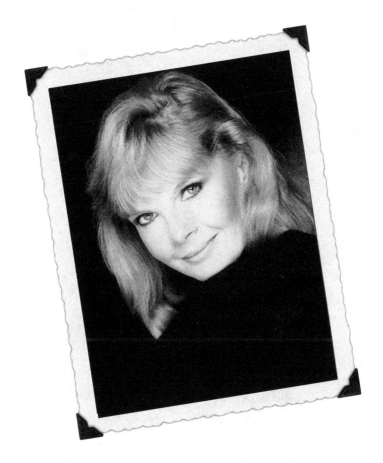

Later on I would learn how to put a happy face before any camera.

6

Losing Control

DECEMBER 1991

This past year was a blur. My life was now built around my appointments at UCLA and juggling the necessary lies to keep my career going. My medications were anti-inflammatories and pain pills. One to take down the inflammation and pain, the other to mask the pain when it refused to go away. The goal of my doctor was to come up with the right combination of medications to halt my disease. So far, we had not found that combination. If a drug worked to take down inflammation it seemed only a matter of time before my blood work would show warning signs that it was affecting my liver. Seems everything you take into your body is processed by the liver, and some things, especially medicines, can be very toxic. Dr. Kalunian would call and say stop the drugs immediately and switch me to another one. Luckily there were many anti-inflammatories on the market.

The trips to New York continued, the work continued, but it was all different. Everything in my life was now connected to my health. Only nobody knew it.

"Hey, how are you? I've been trying to reach you all day," Shelly asked. I could picture him sitting at his desk in his eighth-floor all-glass office in what's known as the Black Tower at Universal Studios.

"Crazy, that's how my day has been," I answered, slipping off my sneakers without untying the laces and flopping back on the bed at the Essex House hotel in New York. "I have almost all the items pulled for my fashion segment. Spent the entire day running from showroom to showroom and then back to the hotel to meet with my assistants and take stock of where we are," I said.

"You sound tired."

"I'm doing fine," I lied, rubbing the bottoms of my red, puffy feet as I talked. "Of course the producer decided about thirty minutes ago to change the direction. Seems he doesn't want holiday fashionable gifts after all, he now wants outfits to wear to holiday events, so tomorrow we start from zero."

"Remember, Christine, this isn't about you. This is about him. It's control. He needs to feel in control of the segment. Don't take it personally," my wise husband advised.

"You're right," I answered, convincing Shelly but not myself. I knew it was about control, but I couldn't get past the thought that he was just trying to make my life more difficult, or maybe it was just that my life was more difficult now a days. "What about your day?" I asked, changing the focus.

"Great, except you're not here. I have to go to the cancer fund-raiser at the Beverly Hills Hotel tonight, and I dread going without you."

I was actually relieved that I would miss having to get dressed up and take pain pills to get through another black-tie party. Whereas I once looked forward to these events, they now demanded too much of my body. The thought of a hot bath, room service, and crawling into bed early sounded delicious. The addition of even more medications plus pain pills to try to control my flaring RA still played havoc with my stomach, but I had no other options. I wasn't sure what was worse, the nausea or the joint pain. As much as I missed Shelly, I didn't miss concealing from him how sick I really felt. Married twenty months. Five great ones and fifteen pain-filled ones, still a better percentage than a lot of marriages I knew. Even though I tried to hide my pain, I often felt as if Shelly was cheated. He didn't get what he thought he was getting. But then, neither did I. In our business, deals are not always what they seem.

The phone woke me at seven o'clock, New York time, fifteen minutes before the alarm.

"Michael wants you to bring the outfits to the studio this afternoon so he can take a look at them," my segment producer Mary Ann said. Michael was the new executive producer. When I started at *Live* he was an intern, then a production assistant, referred to as a PA, but being very ambitious and close to Regis, he quickly moved up. When the executive producer, Steve Ober—the one who started me doing makeovers for ABC in San Francisco—got the New York job with Regis he quickly brought me to New York to work. Now Steve, frustrated at *Live* still being a local morning show when ABC kept promising him year after year that it was going national, had moved on to produce the new, national *Joan Rivers Show* in Los Angeles and the New York local *Live* top job went to Michael.

Bring the clothes to the studio? I never brought the clothes to the studio until the morning of the show, and I'd been working the *Live with Regis and Kathie Lee* show for more than eight years. Anxiety overwhelmed me as I tried to reply, "But he just changed the direction of my segment last night, and I need the full day to pull new merchandise."

"I know, Christine, but you know how it is; he's decided he wants to see the clothes and make sure he likes them."

Since when did he become a fashion stylist? I silently screamed. What the hell is this about? *Make sure he likes them?*

"Just bring what you can and be here by four o'clock. I'm sorry, but you know there's nothing I can do." I knew it was true; there was nothing she could do. When Michael spoke, everyone jumped. Michael was into control, it was a game we all had to play and only he got to win.

Reaching for my Maalox, I rummaged through my tote to find my assistant list. An assistant list is the names and contact numbers for stylists, gofers, anyone who works to help make a segment go together. There are senior assistants, the ones who become your right arm. After working with them for a while they begin to think like you do and anticipate your every need. They know how to handle makeovers to keep them focused and calm and how to pump up models to get them to perform on a "bad image" day when they were squeezing their cellulite in the dressing room mirror and deciding they were too fat to wear a swimsuit on television, after they had been hired as a "swimsuit model." As my disease progressed I was using more assistants to take some of the workload off my aching shoulders. They are expensive, but a good assistant makes all the difference when it comes to a smooth, calm, and organized segment. Smooth and calm were desperately needed in my life these days. Then there are the gofers, the ones who steam, iron, hem, and make temporary alterations at the last minute, tape the bottoms of shoes so they don't get scuffed when models walk in them, and take off price tags before the show, label them lightly with pencil, and organize them into envelopes so they can easily be identified and reapplied after the show. Every good assistant has a tagger, a little instrument that puts the tags on to look like they have never been removed. We borrow most clothes from manufacturers or major department stores, but many of the stores have a policy where a stylist can borrow as long as a percentage—usually twenty percent of everything borrowed—is purchased. Although this can add to your wardrobe, it also adds to your bottom line of costs. Then there are the last-minute grab-and-buy purchases: the fill-in method when you're desperate for items you need and there's no time to go through the corporate channels and all the paperwork to borrow. By using different credit cards, different stores, and different assistants to do the buying and returning you can get away with it, most of the time. If there are lots of returns we will send an assistant's mother. They never question the mothers; it's the stylish young assistants who often look like they have "stylist" tattooed on their foreheads. Or in a hurry they buy ten necklaces, all from one store, just so I will have a choice, when all I need is one for the model. It always sets off an alarm in the head of the salesperson and they know right away that the customer is a stylist. If the salesperson is cool they will go ahead with the purchase. If they are trying to move up to a management job in the store, they will push the little hidden security button, and a strict enforcer will tell you that you can only buy one or two of the same item. They know what you're up to, and their job is to call you on it. I have never known a stylist to be thrown out of a store or go to jail for over-shopping or returning a pair of Jimmy Choo shoes, but the fear is always in the back of our heads.

Today I was desperate to find Amy, my senior assistant, and the only one who could help me though this last-minute Michael emergency without stressing out.

"I know it's last minute but can you work with me today? Change in direction for my segment, and I'm going to need an extra pair of experienced hands. There's no way I can pull this together with two junior assistants." I neglected to say that I was working at about one third of my normal capacity. I probably needed to tell her about my disease, because we had worked closely for seven years, but every time I thought I was ready my gut told me to keep it to myself. One slip, and my career could be over. Plus, Amy is twenty-three. How could she relate to arthritis?

"Sure, Christine, I'll be at your hotel by ten o'clock."

"Perfect." This would allow me to get my other assistants organized and out into the field before she arrived. They had no idea that everything we worked on for the past few days had been canned.

"I'd like a protein shake and one order of plain wheat toast, dry. Yes, Schwab, room 1608, as soon as possible." I hoped the shake would coat my queasy stomach. I hadn't taken my daily pills yet, and already my insides were agitated.

For the first time I dropped the phone's receiver as I tried to place it back in the cradle, my hands cramping up, twisted and frozen in pain. I slumped to the floor, frustrated tears streaming down my face. As much as I tried, I couldn't ignore that the disease was spreading to my hands. Once only sensitive, now my hands were unable to do many of the necessities of my work. Carrying large groups of hanging garments, picking up small items, opening packages—once-simple tasks were now difficult, sometimes impossible. How could I get through this day? This segment?

The ringing phone startled me back to the moment.

"Good morning, gorgeous," Shelly said in that sleepy, sexy morning voice of his.

Quickly masking my tears, I replied, "Good morning."

"I'm lying here in bed thinking of your great body and wishing you were here to wake me up the right way," he whispered.

"Me too, but I'll be home soon."

"So what's on your agenda today?"

"Work, just waiting for my assistants so we can get started. Michael wants me to bring the clothes to the studio this afternoon so he can make sure he likes them."

"Don't get caught up in this game playing, Christine. This is not about you. Why make it more stressful for yourself? Do you think all Michael does all day is try to figure out how to make your work more difficult? You know the protocol. You have to adjust to him, he doesn't have to adjust to you."

"He was an intern when I started, Shelly. Now all of a sudden he has the big job, and I have to prove myself all over again."

"It's just television. Try to keep it in perspective and hurry home. I miss you."

"I miss you, too. I know you're right, but I'm dealing with so much frustration doing my work right now and then this? I don't deserve this power-play treatment after all the successful segments I've done for the show. Ah, hold on, room service is trying to deliver my breakfast."

"No, you go and eat, you haven't been eating well lately, and I don't want you to get scrawny on me. Love ya, talk tonight." And he was gone, ready to start his busy, long day. Never complaining. I needed to get myself back on track. Negative thoughts were filling my once-positive head.

Flashbacks of past Christmases with my mom, some good and some sad, loomed before me as I looked out my hotel window at Central Park below. Even the horses and carriages taking tourists up and down the streets were decorated with holiday garland. As an adult I always went overboard at Christmas—too many gifts, too many parties, too much food. I had to make it perfect. As a child I didn't have any control over making the holidays perfect. Christmas was a time of feeling left out at my "boarded-out" homes. There were trees and gifts under their trees, but as I snooped at the tags, none of them were ever for me. My mom would have a little tree in her apartment and many gifts under it that were for me, but our Christmastimes were always short, and my gifts needed to stay at her apartment so the other "boarded-out" kids wouldn't take them. I had two lives, the one with my mom that I loved and the one with the families who saw me as a monthly check. One was glamorous and loving, the other cold and unknown. Now as an adult I was once again living two lives, one glamorous and loving with Shelly and the other medically unknown. So much had changed from my childhood and yet, recently, at times it seemed as if nothing had changed.

The holiday outfits passed Michael's "inspection," mostly because he was distracted by a last-minute booking cancellation for the next day's show. Easier than I anticipated.

"If you change the white tuxedo shirt for a black-and-white striped one it'll look better on camera, otherwise I guess it's fine," Michael told me, rushing through the rack of eight holiday outfits.

"I GUESS it's fine . . . I GUESS." Keep *your mouth shut, Christine, you've got the okay, change the shirt and get out of here. This is not about you. Just get back to the hotel and get some rest so you don't look as haggard as you feel on TV tomorrow morning.*

"Will do. See you in the morning," I said as I left the garments hanging on the rolling rack that we would attack with steamers in the dark of the early morning. One shirt to change, really no big deal; it's just control.

Catching a cab from the WABC-TV studios on the west side to Bloomingdale's, the closest department store on the east side, I realized I couldn't do it. I couldn't go to the store and buy a replacement tuxedo shirt. I was depleted. The thought of walking through a department store, putting one throbbing foot in front of the other, overwhelmed me. I had no energy left. I was totally and completely exhausted.

Dialing my cell phone, I reached one of my junior assistants, "Bonnie, I need you to do me a big favor. I need a striped tuxedo shirt, model size, for tomorrow. Yes, you need to get it now, orders from the honcho. Sorry, but I have a major business commitment tonight or I would pick it up myself, and Amy's on overload. See you in the morning, six sharp."

Bonnie didn't need to know about my RA. Something changed when someone knew. I was aware of the way my two sisters watched me. Independently of each other, I could follow their eyes as they looked to see what shoes I was wearing, how my hands looked, and how I got up out of a chair. I was the oldest, so I was always the one to watch over them. Now they were reversing our roles. My middle sister Susan was a former nurse, so her eyes were trained to look for the signs of the disease's advancement. My younger sister Pam would look deep in my eyes as if the secrets to my health were there, waiting for her to evaluate where I was on the health scale. Both of them were now attorneys, and they couldn't help but ask questions: "How are you feeling? Any changes? How are the new meds?" Instead of feeling loved, which is what they intended, I felt trapped, defined by my disease. When I was with them I couldn't be in denial. And having lived a childhood of denial, it was for me, with this disease, the most comfortable place to be. When we were all together I envisioned the way they whispered to each other when I left the room. It only made me feel more self-conscious.

Sometimes, on good mornings when I was alone, I could forget that I was sick. Then I'd be with one of our four kids, Shelly's three and my son, and I saw the way they watched me, asked me how I was doing in that questioning "is there anything wrong" tone of voice that brought it all back home. I was in dire need of those little moments of escape. The times I could forget and feel normal, if even for an hour. The more people who knew, the harder it would be for me to cope. The entertainment world has little tolerance for illness. One slip and I would be labeled "unreliable, sick, defective," as if I had a drug problem. I wasn't a Magic Johnson who could shock and touch the world with his AIDS revelation. Nor was I the beloved Michael J. Fox, who put Parkinson's disease in the spotlight. I dealt with my illness more like Princess Di with her bulimia or Uma Thurman with her depression—I hid it. Today Jessica Alba talks openly about her battle with anorexia and Christina Applegate deals with her breast cancer in front of the media. That's now, and this was then.

"Change of plans, just drop me at the Essex House," I told the cab driver.

"Will you be needing a cab tonight?"

"No, not tonight."

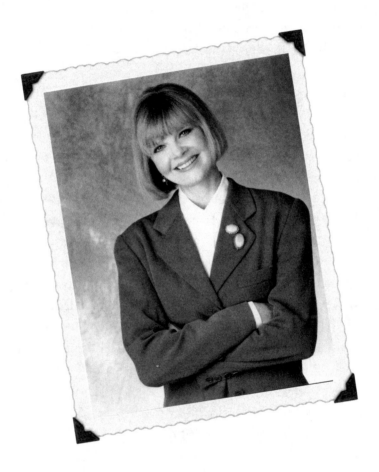

This is my author photo for my first book cover where I used all of my beauty expertise to try to hide my steroid induced "moon face."

7

Playing with Fire

"Everything's in place. We just need Michael to confirm which couples he likes," I told my producer on the phone at *Live*, sitting at my piled-high desk in my condo, looking out at the sunshine-drenched Hollywood Hills. "We were one week away from our weeklong "Light Your Fire Makeovers" and still no decision from our executive producer, Michael, on which five couples would be chosen. He'd let the finalists' folders sit on his desk for more than a week. "I can't get him to concentrate," my producer told me, apologizing for what we both knew she could not control.

This was nothing new. Michael always liked to work on deadline.

"This is New York. Everything's at your disposal. Anything's possible," he told me over and over as he made the last-minute demands that drove me and everyone who worked for him totally crazy. He was right. People changed their lives in order to make a plane the next day to come to New York and be on TV. Stores rearranged their schedules to accommodate our needs, and salons clamored to have the opportunity to work with us. I, of course, adapted. Once anxious to have everything locked down and organized, I now went with the flow, knowing, like Michael, it would somehow work out. If we alienated a few people along the way, Michael didn't care. He taught me it was not only okay but also to be expected. The rationale? It was always the same. We were, after all, the top-rated morning show on television.

Only now, my nervous system was revved. After so many changes in my rheumatoid arthritis medications, searching for the combination that would give me a respite, prednisone, the magical yet dangerous steroid, was what helped me through the times when nothing else would. The type of steroids I took are called corticosteroids. They are very different from the anabolic steroids that athletes use to develop muscle. If I was in desperate pain, a visit to UCLA for an IV of steroids took it away immediately. If I woke up on a morning when I had to do television and my joints were so sore I couldn't walk, a high dosage of steroids limbered me up. Instant relief. They took the inflammation down like nothing else could. They took the pain away, but not without a price, and the more I took them the higher the price became. I never asked about the side effects. I didn't want to know. I only wanted relief. If steroids were often the only thing that worked, and a higher dosage meant more relief, I was all for it. I would deal with any side effects when I felt better. When you're in pain, side effects become secondary to relief. Steroids also made me eat everything in sight, stare at the ceiling when I needed to sleep, and become an overall jittery, nervous wreck. My blood pressure would soar, but my joints felt like new. Steroids put my body into overdrive, 24/7. They were an out-of-body experience, but at least my pain was somewhat manageable, even though the drugs made the other parts of my life spin out of control.

Looking back I understand why I was on steroids. A high dosage would immediately relieve the inflammation in my body when everything else failed. Other times a lower dosage over a longer period of time would do the trick. A frantic call to Dr. Kalunian to say I couldn't walk and I had to attend an awards show, do a television segment, or participate in an industry fund-raiser made it an easy decision for him. Actually, steroids were the only decision, the only relief at these last-minute emergencies. Instant relief, the Band-Aid when I needed a reprieve. I was in such desperate need of being able to function that I never stopped to ask about the long-term side effects. Denial. My childhood of denial now became a tool of my adult existence. Relief was all I cared about at the time. I didn't know what the future held. Pain made me deal with the present. Now I know there was a penalty for the quick fix. I didn't always have to pay right away, but there was no doubt that my charges were accumulating, usually with interest. The immediate charges: instant weight gain and a moon-shaped face. I was worried I was beginning to look like my own "before" picture. Long-term charges: loss of calcium to my bones that caused osteoporosis, and some heart, kidney, and liver issues. Would I take prednisone again? Only if it was an absolute last resort. Do I regret taking it? I didn't have a choice. At the time, my focus was on living as normally as possible, and there was really no other option.

I had a new empathy for people who ate too much. Before steroids I liked food but didn't live for it. Now when a waiter placed the breadbasket on the table I could hardly wait to dig in. I stopped at the 7-Eleven for a Coke and chips on my way to a meeting. I carried not one, but three protein bars in my bag. Sometimes I would even indulge in a Snickers or Reese's Peanut Butter Cup. I was always either thinking about food or eating it. And it showed. I had gained more than twenty pounds and my joints were still too sore to exercise, and unlike today's protocol of keeping joints moving, then the theory was to rest your joints so as to not aggravate them. Today exercise is seen as a treatment, a way to keep the joints moving. My normal size six had changed to a size ten in a month's time. In three months I feared I could be playing for the Dallas Cowboys. Size ten was a nice average size, of course, unless you happened to work in television, and worse yet, in fashion.

Over dinner at California Pizza Kitchen, as I was dipping my bread into golden puddles of rich olive oil, Shelly looked over at me "Are you up for this trip to New York? You don't seem to be doing well."

"I'll be fine. This cough is nothing, just irritating."

"I wasn't referring to just the cough. You're having such a hard time walking."

"Only sometimes. I'm really doing better on this new combination of drugs," I said, devouring my barbecue chicken pizza, my fingers coated in savory, sweet sauce.

"You really don't have to work, Christine. Why don't you take some time off and concentrate on your health? You can always pick up where you left off in the business."

"That's not even a consideration. I'm not a giant in the industry like you. I'm easily replaced. I've worked too hard and long to get where I am to give it away."

"You underestimate yourself. You're great at what you do," Shelly said looking at my empty pizza pan. "Here, have some of my chopped salad. I had a big lunch."

"As long as I'm working. If I stop, no one will remember my name. I have a lot of things I need to accomplish, and giving in to my disease isn't one of them."

"I'm not saying give in, I'm asking you to make it your priority."

"I will never make this my priority. For me that's giving in to the disease," I said, scraping my fork across Shelly's plate to finish the last morsel of his salad.

"What happened to that teddy you used to wear?" my husband asked, lying naked as I crawled into bed wearing my Calvin Klein flannel pajama bottoms and a white long-sleeved T-shirt. I blew out a few of the lavender-scented candles to dim the light.

"It's just so cold," I answered, kissing his neck, hoping to divert his attention away from my flannels. "I'm saving it for summer." After a few more nibbles on his torso he forgot about the flannels. For a man who loved "thin," he had not made any comments on my weight gain. I no longer paraded around naked and managed to light fewer candles and wrap an oversized bath towel around my body after a shower instead of a skimpy one. I also changed many of my slim pants and skirts for roomier, man-tailored ones. Being a fashion stylist helped when you were trying to conceal rapid weight gain. With my steroid-energized, high-speed state, I was wide awake and ready to play at night. Sex was a good distraction from pain and weight.

The one thing I couldn't control or conceal was the weight gain in my face. My once angular jawline was now rounded into what doctors referred to as a "moon face," a puffy, swollen look that is different from a weight gain. It's more like an allergic reaction that swells the face because of the high dosage of steroids. Once the steroids are out of the body, the swelling goes down. This was one of the many side effects of long-term or high dosages of steroids about which they neglected to tell me or I chose not to hear when I was in desperate need of relief. I modified my hairstyle to a short, full-banged bob that helped cover up a little, but unlike my body, which I could fashionably hide, my face gave me away. I was dreading going to New York the next week. I had to come up with a good story if anyone said anything.

"Okay, Michael has picked our five couples. I'll have them to you today so you can call and notify the winners." My producer, relieved to have the choices made, called me early in the morning, the week before we began work.

We were cutting it close. I would fly to New York the next day and work on Couple No. 1 the following day, Friday, in order to have them ready for Monday's show. We would take their "before" picture in the studio right after the live show on Friday. Then it would be a day of shopping and hair. With the first couple I would have the luxury of having Saturday in case we needed a little more time. Once the week got going I had exactly twenty-four hours to complete each couple. In addition,

Michael wanted them separated once the makeover began. We needed the camera to catch the incredible look of surprise as they saw each other made over for the first time in front of five million television viewers. It was great television, especially if we picked couples who genuinely liked each other. Having only interviewed them by phone, it wasn't always easy to discern their relationship, but now with years of practice I knew the questions that revealed their personalities and how they felt about each other—most of the time.

"Have you ever done anything that might come up on air and embarrass you or the show?" I would ask. If they took too long to answer I knew we needed to move on to another interview.

"Let's touch base at the end of the day," my producer said, as relieved as I was that we were finally organized and ready. It wasn't easy getting Michael to focus. I was glad that she was the one following him around the office trying to get a decision, and I was safely tucked away on the West Coast knowing that it would get done.

That afternoon I pulled into the UCLA parking structure off Westwood Boulevard. Inside the garage, my windows up tight and doors locked against the outside, I leaned my head back against the headrest and looked out at the hectic hospital activity all around me. Inside my car I felt protected in my own environment. I knew where I was. Maybe it wasn't always a good place, but I had learned how to deal. Another layer of cover-up, and I could handle almost anything.

The medical building and its doctors loomed. Waiting, once again, to give me news about my health, sometimes good, more often not. Most of my life I had been able to keep the bad from penetrating my cocoon of denial. Even my childhood foster families weren't able to infiltrate my cocoon completely. But RA was different; it worked from the inside out. Nothing could protect me from RA, from what news might await me in this building. With a deep breath I slowly and reluctantly left the safety of my car and walked toward the forbidding double doors and to the doctors who held my fate. Powerless. In this medical environment I was powerless.

I had been on a new drug, methotrexate, since October, and my doctor was slowly increasing the dosage as he tried to taper me off the steroids. When I first read about methotrexate, the information overwhelmed me. Methotrexate was described as a drug that inhibits the folate pathway, which inhibits inflammation. It is actually the most powerful and toxic medication to reduce inflammation by blocking the folate pathway. It was developed to treat leukemia with side effects that were long and intense. Nausea, abdominal distress, chills, fever, dizziness, fatigue, mood alterations—I had to stop reading. After two years of trying different medicines that either didn't work on my joint pain or set off alarms with negative lab results, I had now entered the second phase of treatment, and with it the stronger, more toxic drugs. I didn't have a choice. For me, rheumatoid arthritis was a gathering of disease inside my body, building up its forces daily, planning attacks on different joints. Osteoarthritis is a more common disease that almost everyone gets as they age from normal wear and tear on their bodies. Athletes get osteoarthritis at a much younger age because their sports activities wear down their joints. When a joint wears out today, often they can be replaced, or medications given to ease the discomfort. We always hear people say they can tell if it's going to rain because their arthritis kicks in. It may be an old wives tale, but osteoarthritis is affected by damp weather, making many sufferers head to the deserts in the winter months for relief. Rheumatoid arthritis is a totally different animal. It's under the immune deficiency umbrella like lupus or scleroderma. In a healthy body the immune system fights off infections and disease. In an immune-deficient body this system breaks down, and the body not only attacks itself but also is more vulnerable to other outside germs such as colds, flu, and allergies. We use the term arthritis loosely, but in reality the difference between osteoarthritis and rheuma-toid arthritis is huge. They are both painful and do damage, but rheumatoid is the lion to osteo's lamb.

Now ready to move on to stronger drugs out of necessity, I convinced myself that if methotrexate could halt an attack, I was ready. With each assault my joints suffered more deterioration. Lately, the steroids offered less and less relief and more and more complications. I could no longer depend on the steroids alone to be my emergency fix. What would I do when I had to be on television and could barely move? I hoped methotrexate was my new answer.

During a recent appointment with my family doctor I men-tioned the addition of methotrexate to my drug therapy, and instead of sharing in my excitement, he furrowed his brows.

"That's a powerful drug, and with your new tendency toward bronchial problems you need to think twice about taking it," he warned. "It also decreases your resistance to infection."

Over the past two years I had become more focused on pain relief than side effects. I was desperate for anything that worked, and so far nothing did. Every now and again, I took a step back and realized how crazy it all must have looked from the outside. Chronic pain and desperation made me willing to do just about anything. I convinced Dr. Kalunian that I must be able to con-tinue my life as normally as possible. So I went from drug to drug, adjustment to adjustment, searching for the combination that would put me in remission. Dr. Kalunian never gave up hope; he believed it was out there. Having tried so many drugs already, I was not so sure. All I knew was I had to get off steroids. I needed to lose this extra weight and have the shape of my face return to normal. I wanted to feel in control of my life and my body, instead of watching both spin faster and faster out of my grasp.

Spinning out of control as an adult always brought me back to my childhood, when I had absolutely no control. I only wanted to live with my mom. Her reply to that was that it was impossible because of her irregular hours at work. Television wasn't as integrated with nontraditional families then as it is now, so I had no way of knowing that other single mothers made working and raising a child doable. Reluctantly I took her word for boarding out being the only solution and yearned for the day when we could be together. My mom's answer to everything was that my "boarded homes" kept me clean and neat. She was so proud that she had finally taught Margie the "right" way to fix my hair. In my mom's eyes, my life at Margie's was improving. I think good grooming was really important to her because she made up for her lack of education by being beautiful, and that was always her entrée to work and men. Besides, she would say, "We get to see each other and have fun when I'm not working, don't we, Chrissie?"

Now I understand with the help of therapy and time that it was normal to feel isolated and alone without my mom. I was a powerless child living in a house where I didn't belong. My childlike solution was that maybe, just maybe, if my mom thought my foster homes weren't keeping me clean or neat enough, she would let me live with her. But it was my withdrawal and depression, reported by the school principal a few years later, that finally made my mom see that her solution, even with good hair, was not working.

Now, at UCLA, and taking the combination of steroids and methotrexate, my lab results came back okay. I was still anemic, which accounted for my light-headedness. There was some fluid buildup on one elbow that Dr. Kalunian aspirated with a long needle that once would have made me faint. A little dry cough that I hardly noticed, but we'd keep an eye on it. Plane travel played havoc with my joints and my respiratory tract, and I seemed to always be on an airplane.

"I need to get through the next ten days. I have five days of live TV work. Just get me through this next period and then we can adjust," I pleaded. It was a plea Dr. Kalunian heard over and over, every time my schedule went into overdrive.

"That means we can't start taking the steroids down until you get home," Dr. Kalunian said.

"But all of this weight and I can't sleep at night. I am wound like a top. I feel like I'm spinning all the time."

"Christine, the only way I can control your disease right now is with the combination of steroids and methotrexate. It's working pretty well, so let's not fool around until you're over this intense work period," Kalunian advised. I knew he was right. I could always shop for some new, looser dresses in New York while I worked on the makeovers. Something that fashionably hid my body. Here was an ironic advantage of working in an industry that didn't tolerate weight gain: I was remarkably adept at camouflaging it.

In the teddy Shelly loved, now stretched almost to the breaking point over my swollen body, and only one candle burning on my bedside table, we said our romantic good-byes on Wednesday night. Most of the time Shelly arranged his schedule so he could come to New York when I worked, and I did the same when he had to travel, but this time he had to be in Los Angeles, and we would be apart for eight days.

"Let's stand in front of the mirror, I want to remember you in this teddy all week," my aroused husband whispered, referring to the mirrored closet doors in our bedroom. I didn't want to stand in front of any mirror, even in the dim light, and reveal how tight the teddy looked. With some playful distraction he forgot all about his request.

Right before I closed my eyes to go to sleep I looked over at my bedside table, trying in the dark to locate my small round stone with the word "Believe" etched on it. I knew it was there, nestled somewhere between all the stacked books and candles. It was the last thing I looked at before going to sleep. I had placed more of these stones `around the house: in the bathroom where

I did my makeup, in the kitchen where I cooked and now ate everything in sight, on my desk where I organized segments and worked at my computer. I kept a smaller version in my purse and my travel luggage. They were a constant reminder that if I believed I would be okay, I would. And lately, as so many medicines had failed me, I needed daily reminding. On this night, I moved it closer to the edge of the table so I could reach over and run my aching fingers over the etched word "Believe." On this night with a busy workweek ahead of me, I needed extra belief.

New York was not easy in February, especially when I was on a demanding, tight schedule with no room for error. The daily weather report informed me how easy or difficult my day would be. That particular Friday, the first day of making over a couple for Monday's show, the prediction was for snow in the early afternoon. Snow meant problems. A few years back a storm hit New York during a week of makeovers, and the city shut down. Literally. Offices closed, people were sent home, and car services were called back to their headquarters. I had to beg and plead to keep our driver as we crawled through the traffic-jammed city as everyone fought to get out. I had no choice then and no choice this day. Experience had taught me to have two assistants and two cars lined up for every day during the bad-weather months. Don't take chances; there was no time for emergencies. The logistical problems we had on a good day were staggering. This was my schedule:

Nine o'clock A.M: Met Couple No.1 at the studio. In their early thirties, they had great, untapped potential. Both had pale skin and mousy-colored brown virgin hair. The wife told me during the phone interview that she cuts their hair and, in person, I would have guessed it. I talked with them about our itinerary and hyped them about the experience. They already agreed before confirming their trip that I could do "anything" I needed for their makeover. People always agree on the phone; in person, it was another thing.

Ten fifteen A.M: "Before" shot was taken of the couple together and then individually. No makeup or smiling allowed. Oh, and I encouraged them to wear dull colors or busy prints. Basically, I was looking for the worst imaginable Sears photo shoot. My assistant Amy would take the husband to Bloomingdale's to start pulling clothes while I took the wife to the salon to start on her hair, where my second assistant Bonnie would help. Fortunately, the couple resembled the picture they sent in with their nomination letter except for the wife's front chipped tooth, which had to be fixed.

"Amy, call Dr. Rosenthal and see if we can stop by on our way to the salon. I think we need a bonding on the front teeth." I stalled while Amy called, revving up our couple for their day and reiterating once again the importance of their not seeing each other or talking about what makeover changes we made that day. We needed the big reveal on camera. They were booked at separate hotels and would be separated in the dressing rooms at the studio but, bottom line, we depended on them playing along. Some did, but others loved the mischievousness of hooking up the night before and trying out their new looks on each other.

"Rosenthal is okay for the bonding, no problem," Amy said. Off we went in different cars, different directions and began our intense day of makeovers.

Ten thirty A.M: Amy took the husband shopping. My second assistant Bonnie and I took the wife to Dr. Rosenthal's office for a quick consultation.

Eleven fifteen A.M: Teeth impressions made, Bonnie and I arrived at the salon for hair consultation.

Eleven forty-five A.M: Consultation completed and work started on the wife. I left for Bloomingdale's to see what clothing Amy pulled for the husband. Made a few minor changes. He had a contemporary outfit of cargo-pocketed cords, a high-cut V-neck cashmere sweater, and sports coat. A pair of sunglasses, even though it was February, would make a dramatic camera impression in the morning. I made an excuse about needing to work on the schedule in order to sit in the dressing room and give my aching body a rest. Amy took the husband to lunch in Bloomingdale's and then would pick out shoes while we stalled the return to the salon until his wife was done and moved out of his sight. I headed back to the salon, amazed that it was only noon and my knees and feet were already screaming.

Twelve thirty P.M: I arrived at the salon and saw that the wife's hair color was still a little drab. Television lights and cameras soaked up color, and I needed that wow factor when she walked out for the reveal.

"Let's add some baby-blond highlights right in front to pop her color," I said, trying to hide my disappointment. Bonnie informed me privately that she had already had three color applications to get where they were now and our makeover was getting a little nervous. It was my job to assure her that all was well and she only needed a minor tweaking, nothing damaging, in order to reach perfection. A hand on her shoulder as I talked helped her feel my confidence and she was once again happy and eager to see her new cut and style and hit the stores for her head-to-toe outfit. She was a sweet, shy lady who never invested any time or money in her looks. She hardly smiled, probably because of the chip in her tooth.

This was why I loved working on makeovers. The potential to change someone's life for the better inspired me. To show someone they were more than they thought, that they could rise above anything, took me back to my childhood where I never felt worthy. Because my mother boarded me in other people's homes, I was always the outsider, the unwanted one. A weekend several times a month with my mother wasn't enough to give me a feeling of self-worth. And so with each makeover, right before the cameras went on, I looked at where I was and what I'd accomplished and remembered where I came from and I knew I was meant to do this work.

One o'clock P.M: We ordered lunch and ate in the salon amid plastic capes, hair color, and cut hair on the floor as the work continued. By now I was used to a few hair clippings in my salad.

One thirty P.M: The color was perfect. We proceeded with the cut. Amy called to inform me that our husband was well dressed and well fed and ready for the salon. I told her to take him for a coffee and plan to arrive at the salon by Two thirty.

"Amy, will you stop on your way back to the salon and buy me a chocolate milk?" I had to coat my stomach so I could take a pain pill to help me survive the rest of the day. Amy knew to call before entering the salon to make sure we had the wife hidden. We couldn't take any chance of passing in the elevator or on the street.

Two thirty P.M: Hair completed, Bonnie took the wife to Bloomingdale's to shop. I would meet them as soon as I started the husband in the salon.

Three o'clock P.M: Husband arrived, we consulted and decided his mustache needed to come off since his hair was short and not easily changed. He reluctantly agreed once I told him we were going to put a few sun-inspired highlights in his brown hair. "Put a little self-tanner on his face to blend the pale skin where his mustache was," I told one of the salon assistants, handing them a tube of instant tanner I always carried in my work tote. Men loved the personal attention even though they didn't often like to admit it. All was under control at the salon, so I headed back to Bloomingdale's to see how our wardrobe was coming together, calling Rosenthal's office to update them on our time schedule. They needed us at the office as soon as possible to start the bonding process. In the cab I gulped my chocolate milk with my pain pill.

Three fifteen P.M: On the fourth floor of Bloomingdale's, I found a distraught and slightly hostile wife. Amy had picked out a Jackie-O-inspired sleeveless shift dress in a chocolate brown with a pink band at the hem. Stunning, but our makeover hated it.

"I look frumpy, I want to look sexy," she complained, glaring at the evil Amy, who insisted she looked incredible.

"She wants something with cleavage," Amy explained, taking me aside. She informed me that four children have taken their toll on her cleavage and it was best to cover it up. My only chance to get past this was to appear to give in.

"If she wants cleavage, let's try cleavage," I said, as I made my way through the racks looking for low-cut items. Armed with several it was back to the dressing rooms, where a happy makeover candidate thought I was taking her side.

"Try these on one at a time and come out and show me, even if you don't like it, just to give me an idea of what works and what doesn't," I said. I whispered to Amy, "Don't comment when she comes out."

With each change our makeover grew more excited, loving the revealing clothes. Only problem was that they revealed way too much. "I think we can find something better, this one hides your legs. You have incredible legs, let's show them off," I said. Slowly I convinced her that her legs were her best assets, not her breasts. "Would you mind trying the brown dress on for me just one more time, I need to see the shape so we know where to go from here" and she willingly agreed. I had won her over.

"Oh my God, you look incredible. This dress makes you look taller and slimmer and sexier than any of the other outfits. If we add a pair of stilettos, your husband will go crazy. You look sexier than Michelle Pfeiffer" (recalling a name she mentioned to me on the phone when I asked her what celebrities she liked). She agreed. Amy quickly brought me a pair of high, high pumps, and it was a done deal. She looked and felt hot. Sizzling actually.

"Now for the fun part, accessorizing. I want to find the sexiest underwear in the store and some chandelier earrings that will sparkle and swing as you walk out to greet your adorable husband." By four forty-five we were finished. Mission completed, so far. My pain pill was finally working, allowing my feet to work even though my stomach ached from being overly medicated.

Five fifteen P.M: The snow had arrived, but thankfully it was a light flurry. Most of it melted before it hit the ground. Amy took our makeover to Dr. Rosenthal's office for bonding, and I returned to the salon to check her husband's progress. He was in the midst of getting a manicure and pedicure to fill time waiting for my return. He looked wonderful. It never ceased to amaze me what a stylish haircut, a little hair color, and some instant tanner would do. The color change was lighter than I anticipated, but very Brad Pitt, and it suited him. The self-tanner was just enough color to make him look as if he spent the day by the pool. He loved the attention, especially the young manicurist, fluttering her long lashes and bending over his cuticles with half her breasts hanging out. Not wanting to take away from his obvious enjoyment, I quickly complimented him.

"You look great, wait until your wife sees you on Monday. Now remember, no contact over the weekend. Bonnie will get you back to your hotel and pick you up at six thirty Monday morning. I'll check in with you on Sunday. Wash your hair and shave Monday before we pick you up. We'll bring your new clothes. Have a relaxing weekend." I'm sure he was thinking of her all weekend. The Friday couple's makeover was always the most difficult because they have to be in the city on their own and separated until Monday.

Six o'clock P.M: I arrived at Rosenthal's office. Bonding was in progress, so I had a few minutes to relax and browse through magazines in the waiting room. My chest was slightly congested, but my body was trying to figure it all out, conflicted between pain pill sedation and steroid-induced hyperactivity.

"Amy, will you get me a chamomile tea?" In the quiet after-hours of the office I tried to unwind with a magazine, but my mind raced, plotting out tomorrow's activities. The week had only just begun.

"I need to see her in the office tomorrow," Dr. Rosenthal informed me, coming into the empty waiting room. "She's disappointed, because she can't wait to see her new teeth, but she's also tired and not tolerating the bonding well tonight. I would rather finish up after she gets a good night's rest. Can you have her here at ten o'clock A.M?"

"Of course, she probably didn't get any sleep the night before flying to New York, and with all the excitement of today it's a good idea to finish tomorrow."

Amy arrived back with my tea, and I asked about her availability Saturday. "I'm going to a wedding in New Jersey."

"Ah, well, I'll give Bonnie a call," I said.

"Bonnie's invited to the same wedding" Amy said. I knew it would be me and my makeover bonding, literally, for most of Saturday.

Seven thirty P.M: We all left Rosenthal's office in a heavier snow that now blanketed the city. My makeover was exhausted. "Why don't you order room service and just relax tonight? I'll pick you up at Nine thirty in the morning," I said as we made the first cab stop at her hotel.

Eight fifteen P.M: I walked through the doors of my hotel, starving and exhausted. I had no plans for the weekend that didn't include work. In the city that never stopped, I needed to stop and conserve my energy.

At the show on Monday morning we struggled to keep the makeover couple separated. Their excitement levels were off the charts, and between the awareness of being on national television and the anticipation of seeing each other, many trips to the bathrooms were necessary. The studio's men's and women's bathrooms were right next to one other, so I had Bonnie stand guard for fear that they would bump into each other. The make-overs' energy filled our small dressing room, affecting everyone from the hair designers to the assistants. When the stage manager came to take us to the stage, it all fell into place. A calmness came over everyone. From the dentist to the makeup artist, the camaraderie of our work was now standing in front of us, beaming, her hands clasped tightly together to keep them from shaking. The theme music swelled, and off we went. It was show-time.

Regis introduced the husband first and the audience went wild. After I explained what was done to our makeover guy we took a commercial break. I didn't think he'd make it until his wife came out, he was so eager to see her.

"Did you change her hair color?" the husband asked.

"You'll see in a minute," I answered, trying to calm him down and get him to stand on the taped X on the floor, his camera mark.

"Do you think she'll like my look?" he asked.

"She'll love it," I answered, adjusting his sweater, which he had somehow twisted on his torso.

"Are you ready to see the missus?" Regis asked.

"Yup," was all he could get out. While the cameras rolled he had become tongue-tied.

"Well, here—she—is," Regis said, indicating the side cur-tains where she appeared.

We didn't need to say any more. Love took over, and said it all. He rushed over to his wife, put his arms around her, and gazed into her face with the look every woman dreamed of.

"You're beautiful," he said, not taking his eyes off her. For the first time she smiled ear to ear, revealing her new bonded teeth.

"You're gorgeous, I love your hair," she said, running her fingers through it. They kissed a soap opera kiss. Regis tried to tear them apart, but they were lost in their own world. This is what made my work magical. Not only did they look amazing, but fixing the chipped tooth had transformed a shy wife into a confident woman. Her smile said it all.

For those few incredible minutes on television I was pain free. I was not an abandoned child. I was not a sick UCLA patient. I was an accomplished woman.

I didn't get to talk about her makeover on TV—there wasn't any reason to. Their actions told the story of a young couple who had discovered each other once again. We went to commercial break. I walked back to the dressing room to clean up and organize for Couple No.2, who waited in the green room for their makeover for tomorrow's show. The process was about to start all over again and I couldn't miss a beat, especially since Michael was watching.

"Are you taking steroids?" Michael asked me as I stood by his desk, trying to confirm future projects. Surprised, I didn't know how to answer.

"What made you say that?" was all I could come up with at the moment.

"My friend was on steroids, and her face looked swollen like yours," he said, making me feel totally self-conscious.

"I've got a lung infection. Doctor thinks it's from so much airplane travel. He put me on prednisone to clear it up." It took all of my discipline not to wheeze or cough while I talked.

Michael, being Michael, shrugged his shoulders and started scrolling through his e-mails, dismissing me in his usual manner. I left without a future TV date, which was not unusual. Michael liked to keep talent off guard, his power play in position.

"I'll call you about a date," he said. Translated, I'm busy, this is not a priority, you'll chase me down. It was the dance we danced, at his convenience. I left powerless and frightened that my cover-up was wearing thin. I wasn't sure if I felt so overwhelmed because of his probing questions or because of my unending bronchial problems.

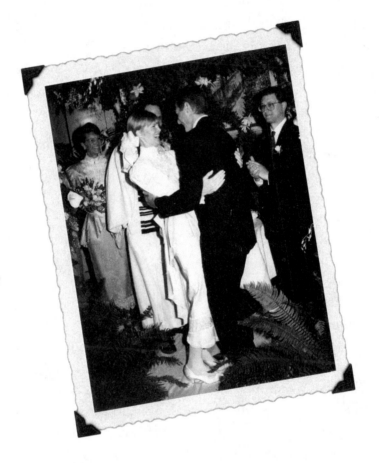

My health issues surfaced shortly after one of the happiest days of my life.

8

Pepperoni Pizza at Cedars

Two weeks after the Light My Fire Makeovers, when I was safely back at home, my health took a major turn for the worse.

Dr. Gordon, my pulmonary specialist, looked at me over the top of his tortoiseshell half glasses as I sat on the exam table and said, "I have to put you in the hospital, Christine. I know how you feel about this, but your fever keeps spiking, and despite two weeks of various broad-spectrum antibiotics you're getting worse. I want you to check into Cedars—today." Up until then I had been able to convince him I was better off at home, but not today. Today I knew he was not giving me a choice. I looked around at the dreary room. I fit in perfectly.

"We need to find out what's causing the fever and get a further evaluation. I'll call the hospital, make the arrangements, and set up the tests we need. Go home and pack your bag."

I was devastated. The hospital. We were due to travel to Chicago next week. I was working on a book proposal. I had six upcoming television segments to put together. I convinced myself that working in freezing temperatures a few weeks ago in New York caused this setback. Sloshing through melted snow puddles would make anyone sick. Wouldn't it?

I loved snow as an adult because I never saw it as a child. Living in Los Angeles, the closest snow was a few hours away by car, and, as a "boarded-out" child, the only trips I took in cars were when my mom picked me up. People who take in kids for money take them in to live in their house, eat at their table, and sleep in their beds. It never included any trips to markets, movies, or even the local snow. That line was firmly drawn between boarders and family.

One day out of frustration at not being able to go to the local mountains with Margie and Bill and their kids, I asked the sitter to call my mom and tell her, but when I couldn't remember her phone number that put an end to that. "Maybe she'll call you," the sitter said.

But I knew my mom wouldn't call. She never called to talk to me because I would always cry and ask her to come pick me up.

"You make me so sad, Chrissie. You know I have to work. I come pick you up whenever I can," my mom tried to explain.

"Hi love, do you have a sec?" I wheezed into the phone to Shelly later that afternoon, cuddled up in my afghan on the cozy chenille den sofa watching an old Diane Keaton movie. Watching television in the daytime should have made me realize just how bad things were. I never sat still long enough to watch daytime TV before.

"I was just getting ready to call you. How did it go at the doctor's this morning?" Shelly asked.

"Not so good. I have to check into Cedars for tests."

"Well maybe now he can get to the bottom of this, find out why you're not getting better. I'm going to clear my calendar, and I'll pick you up after your tests and take you to Orso." I pictured Shelly hurriedly writing notes for his assistant on what to reschedule.

"No dinner, I have to stay in the hospital for a few days, just until they get the test results."

"Well then I'll bring Orso to you," Shelly said. "I'll be there at seven o'clock with your spaghetti all'arrabbiata."

I gathered my toiletries, clothes, pajamas, robe, Filofax, and work folders. I planned on making my business calls from the hospital; no one would need to know that I was not in my home.

My room was small and sterile and smelled of Lysol. I placed a few family pictures on the bedside table: my son Erik in his USC cap and gown, my stepdaughter Kerry, the television publicist, and my stepson Kyle sitting under a big shade tree with one of Kyle's rescue dogs poised between them. A group shot of me with my half sisters, Pam and Susan, arms lovingly intertwined, and of course Shelly, sitting on a chair in his office looking distinguished and presidential. I didn't even think to bring a picture of my mom. She knew I was going into the hospital, but I knew she would never call to check up on me, and I didn't need a picture to remind me of that. With my mom the emphasis was never on how to be a good person, but on how to clean my room. It wasn't about using proper English but on choosing the right wardrobe colors. Not on good grades but on good hair. Studying wasn't important to her—she only had an eighth-grade education. Her priorities were teaching me to stand in the first ballet position for a photo and the values of using a good tingling facial masque to make my skin glow. Without knowing it at the time, she prepared me for my television fashion career. She never prepared me for the realities of life, let alone the strength I'd need to deal with disease.

By the time I unpacked and changed into the hospital gown the evening lights were starting to go on in the city below me. I felt out of breath and light-headed. I should have been used to that feeling of needing to sit down to catch my breath, but it was so against my nature that it still surprised me even after two years of living with RA.

"What are you doing out of bed?" the nurse asked as she rolled the IV bottle into my room.

"Doctor-ordered IV of erythromycin. Should make you feel better," She reached for my arm with her elastic band and needle.

"It's freezing in here."

"It's you, your fever is 102, and you're shivering. We need to get that down," the nurse told me, taping the needle firmly into my arm.

The noises of the hospital—visitors talking in the hallways, a floor waxer polishing outside my door, carts moving from place to place—all kept me from sleep. I decided to accomplish something and called my assistant Amy.

"Amy, hi. Look, I've got lots going on right now and was wondering if you could take over some of the fashion-segment calls. Mostly showrooms and manufacturers to see if they have what I need." On my last trip to New York I finally had to tell Amy about my RA. I knew from the way she looked at me and the things I would ask her to help with, things I would normally do, that she was aware something wasn't right. Because she was young and didn't know about RA, she just listened and assured me she would be there for me and keep everything under wraps.

"Sure, I've got time. Fax me the list of what you're looking for, and I'll start calling tomorrow. You don't sound good, is that cold still bothering you?"

"Yeah, I can't get rid of it. Between the weather in New York, the airplanes, and now all this talking on the phone, I can't seem to shake it. I'll fax you tomorrow and then call you in a day or so, no need for you to track me down." I wanted to hang up quickly before I started coughing again.

"Don't worry about a thing, Christine, just take it easy."

"Thanks, talk to you in a few days," I said in my hoarse voice, as I pulled the hospital blankets up around my trembling body.

Why couldn't I ever stop? Why did I always need to prove myself over and over? I knew the answers. I just didn't want to think about them right now.

The next day Shelly had his assistant fax the information to Amy. She made the necessary business calls, only now I couldn't return her calls because I was too sick. My cough was almost nonstop, making any conversation difficult. And really, at this point I hardly cared about work. I hardly cared about anything.

For four days I lay in the hospital, only getting up to use the bathroom, which was a major ordeal. My outings now consisted of a trip by wheelchair to a testing room and Shelly's nightly visits, which exhausted me. Trying to carry on a conversation made me cough. So he would tell me about his day and I would try to smile and nod, when all I wanted to do was close my eyes and sleep. Morning, noon, and night I was served meals that didn't look or smell appetizing, even by hospital standards. The flowers from Shelly, white daises, my favorites, were of no comfort. I dozed in and out all day and night, irritated by the many interruptions of doctors, nurses, and cleaning people. All I wanted was to be left alone, I didn't want to see or talk to anybody. I couldn't get enough air in my lungs to keep me from wheezing. My cell phone would ring, and I never had the energy nor inclination to see who it was. I didn't care about anything or anyone. I felt as if the life was draining out of me. The nurses would tell me "you'll feel better tomorrow," but I knew they were just trying to hide from me how gravely sick I was.

Four doctors, an infectious disease evaluation, gallium scan, fiber-optic bronchoscopy and endoscopy, and numerous biopsies later, I was worse. Each doctor came into my room with test results, which, except for pneumonia with granulomas, and some anemia, seemed to be normal. So why was I weaker and sicker with every day? Why couldn't I rally myself to care? It wasn't like me to give up, even with a battle this hard and scary.

On the fifth night in the hospital, Shelly decided to surprise me by bringing his daughter Kerry to visit. She was my first visitor other than Shelly because I had specifically requested "no visitors." Kerry, being a publicist in television, didn't take no for an answer. She was sure she could cheer me up. I just wasn't up to being cheered. They arrived after work carrying take-out containers from the Daily Grill.

"Chicken picatta and mashed potatoes with spinach," Kerry gushed in her overenthusiastic manner. "How can anyone look so good in the hospital?" she lied, trying to make me feel better.

One of my all-time favorite meals looked unappealing. Even with all the steroids being pumped into my veins, they couldn't make even that food appetizing. Not tonight. Not in this hospital. I politely moved the food around the paper plate on my bed tray while they hungrily devoured theirs, making way-too-chipper small talk.

I couldn't contribute because it only made me cough. I was so exhausted and uncomfortable all I could think about was when they would leave. After an hour I gave Shelly the look, and he packed up and gave me a kiss. As they walked out, I barely made it to the bathroom to throw up. Their good-natured visit overwhelmed me. I was so weak it was all I could do to crawl back into bed and close my eyes. I didn't know if I would ever leave the hospital.

The next morning the phone rang while the nurse changed my IV.

"Just a minute, she's right here," she said, handing me the phone despite my frantic waving and shaking my head no. "It's your doctor from UCLA," she whispered.

"Christine, Ken Kalunian, I just heard you were at Cedars. What's going on?" I couldn't even answer him. All I could do was cough and cry. I was so glad to hear his friendly, reassuring voice. Dr. Kalunian didn't know it, but over the last year he had become my new best friend.

"It's okay, take it easy. I just want to talk to you. Gordon gave me your test results. When did you stop taking the methotrexate?"

Between coughs and tears I answered, "I'm still taking it." Why would I want to stop? It worked the best of any of the drugs so far. At least my RA was not the problem. I heard a muted gasp over the phone.

"YOU'RE STILL TAKING METHOTREXATE?" he said, almost shouting. "*Does Dr. Gordon know?*"

"We've never talked about the methotrexate."

"But he does know you are taking it, right?"

"Of course, he never liked the idea that I was going on it in the first place, before all of this illness even started."

"Does he know you're taking it in the hospital?"

"I don't know, I hardly see him, it's all specialists, but why would he think I had stopped?" I asked between coughs.

"You MUST stop. I can't believe he hasn't taken you off already. I think most of your problems might be caused by methrotrexate lung poisoning. Some people are allergic, and I think you might be one. I wish I'd known you were sick."

"I never thought to call you because my RA has been doing great, it's all this lung stuff. I never put the two together, and the nurses kept bringing my medications."

"How would you know? Your doctor should have known, or called me earlier." I could tell he was working hard to cover up his agitation.

The healthy me would have been furious. Nobody checking on my medications to see if one of them was causing my severe illness. The normal me would have been angry. If this was the type of care I was getting, I'd have been better off at home where I could sleep without a million interruptions. But this was the sick me, the sickest I had ever been in my life. I didn't have the energy to be anything. I curled up in a fetal position, pulling the covers over my head, and sobbed.

On my sixth day in the hospital, after stopping methotrexate, I started to feel better. Dr. Gordon visited in the afternoon.

"Your tests came back fairly normal except for the nuclear scan. That one lit up your lungs like a Christmas tree. Your biopsies showed an interstitial pneumonitis with granulomas. This is deemed consistent with the diagnosis of methotrexate lung disease. By stopping all antibiotics and methotrexate your condition is improving."

It was still all I could do to keep my eyes open, I was so exhausted. My body seemed to be my own once again, but the fear that RA or the medications to treat RA could make me this sick loomed heavy in my mind. If it could happen once, could it happen again? All I wanted to do was get out of the hospital and back to my life, the one before RA.

"Thanks for the pizza. I can't believe how much I craved a slice of pepperoni," I said to Shelly later that night as we sat side by side on my hospital bed with the Mulberry pizza box on our laps.

"I knew you turned a corner when you asked for a pizza," he said.

"Dr. Gordon said I might be able to come home tomorrow if my fever is still down." I ran my hand through Shelly's hair, the first time I had really touched him in more than a week, the first time I felt like a human being.

It was a beautiful sunny winter day in Los Angeles as Shelly drove me home from Cedars. "Your messages are saved on the phone," Shelly told me over the fifteen-minute ride from the hospital to our condo. It was the first time I thought of messages, work, projects that have been ignored, or unreturned calls. Everything looked so lush and green. People rushed in cars and on sidewalks. The streets seemed busy, so occupied with life. Nobody was wearing hospital greens. Life was bustling. The life I missed. The life I never thought I'd return to. I realized I had given up. I never gave up on my unhappy life as a child, but disease never had been a part of my life as a child or an adult, until now. The power of disease made me shudder even though the sunlight was streaming in through the windshield. As I looked over at my husband, the thought of loss overwhelmed me with sadness. Could I really have given up on my career and my life so easily?

In my work I had always concentrated not on who I was, but on how I could improve. I understood the vulnerability of my job, having seen too many television personalities find out they were replaced by reading a tabloid story or watching the television news. This fear kept me on my toes and looking over my shoulder. The thought of losing my career to this disease was too close to the childhood fears that still haunted me. Three foster homes in six years had left me scared and insecure. Security was not a familiar word in my vocabulary. I had learned about survival, but trust? Trust was beyond my comprehension.

When I first met Shelly it was all about the glitz and glamour. Our pasts were so different, our present paralleled in some ways, but our future became solidified because of our similar values. We both loved to have fun, were passionate to succeed, and, as we grew to know each other, it was our values that enabled us to fall in love. We valued friendship, family, and each other. Slowly I began to learn to trust. Gradually I learned that this was a person who wouldn't abandon me. I knew I could never give up on that.

Our condo looked beautiful. Shelly made the bed, and every dish was washed and put away. The windows opened to my little balcony garden. All my white flowers were in bloom. Without my reminding him, Shelly had taken care of everything. I walked through the rooms, loving each one. Loving being home. But the checkout process had been long and exhausting, so I longed for bed. My own soft pillows and crisp white sheets felt welcoming. No hanging IV bottles. No Lysol. I crawled between the covers, leaving my suitcase packed, my messages saved on the phone, my husband closing the shutters and turning on the sound machine that would dull the city noises so I could rest. I was home.

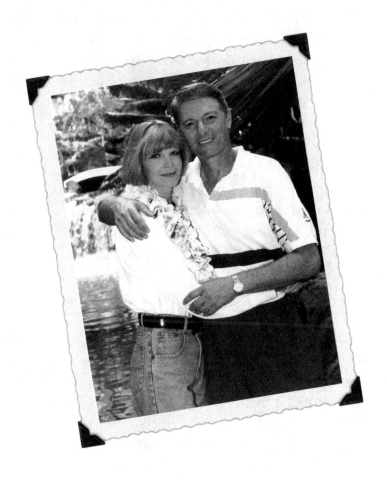

It took steroids to make this Hawaiian trip possible.

9
Running at Steroid Speed

Spring 1992

I had my life back. Or at least my life on pain pills and steroids.

March and April were filled with work. Catching up and moving forward. *Live with Regis, Entertainment Tonight, The Today Show.* My schedule was just the way I liked it, busy and challenging. It felt so good to feel so good.

My lungs were slightly damaged, but considering the condition they were in, they were good. My secret was intact. Everyone believed my story about a lung infection from so much plane travel. I had to guard myself from saying too much. I had the story down so pat that I tended to go overboard with details when in reality no one really cared or listened. They were just glad I was at work.

I was running at above-normal speed. I had endless energy. I barely needed sleep. I felt like superwoman. I was back on steroids, but at a higher dosage. Twenty milligrams a day to be exact. Those magical little pills that masked my arthritis. I never stopped to ask the doctor about more long-term side effects.

"We have to use steroids to take down the methotrexate lung disease, it's the only drug we have to get you back to normal," my pulmonary doctor said as he checked me out of the hospital.

I put the moon face out of my mind. I was only concerned with being alive. I didn't think about every step I took or wince every time I bent my knees or tried to open a car door handle. I could exercise. I had a life back, my life in the high-speed steroid lane.

"What are you doing up at three o'clock in the morning?" my sleepy husband asked me, walking into my office where I had fashion charts and style magazines spread out all over the floor. The room was so brightly lit it looked like daytime. The fireplace blazed against the early morning chill. My cup of coffee was now cold and untouched.

"I couldn't sleep, so I thought I might as well get up and accomplish something. It's so quiet at this hour that I can really get tons done," I said sitting on the floor in the middle of all the clutter.

"But when will you sleep?"

"Don't worry, I'll catch a nap this afternoon," I lied. There was little sleeping at night on steroids; forget about the daytime. "You're edgy," my sister Susan, now working as a full-time nurse in the neonatal department at Harbor General Hospital while going to law school at night, said to me as we enjoyed one of our monthly dinner outings. Even with our crazy, busy schedules, we always made time to be together. Being with my sisters was like medicine for my soul.

"It's the steroids. They're going to start to taper me, but my adrenal gland has to kick in and that takes time." Adrenal glands are the natural producer of steroids that the body requires to function. When they aren't working the body is not getting its needed dosage of natural steroids, making me edgy. Sometimes I felt like I was crawling out of my skin. It was the weirdest feeling. I had to keep moving. I felt jumpy all over. Everything about me seemed hyped—my sensitivity, my reactions, even my skin felt magnified to the slightest touch. But compared to where I had been in the hospital, I only concentrated on the positive.

Usually oblivious to minor things, his head overloaded with work, Shelly had also noticed my quick, irritated reactions. "Jeez, don't jump all over me, we don't have to have the Passover dinner here, we can take the family out this year," Shelly said, trying as usual to find solutions. But I wanted to scream, "Why can't someone else do Passover this year, why always me?" And yet I couldn't scream, I could only apologize for being grumpy. It wouldn't do any good to explain that it wasn't me talking, it was the steroids, my version of the infamous 'roid rages athletes had, minus attacking a trainer with a baseball bat. I looked at my loving husband as he walked away rejected. I hated that I was incapable of being all things to my husband and family. And I worried. Would they be able to accept me as less than perfect? My mom's drive for perfection in appearance was always at the back of my mind. Rheumatoid arthritis took away the ability to be perfect, and not being perfect for me, even as an adult, threatened every fiber of my being.

"Great, Christine, your adrenal gland is finally kicking in, we can start tapering the steroids," Dr. Kalunian announced the following week at my UCLA visit. Between the sun shining through the wooden blinds and his smile, I knew this was a major breakthrough. "We'll take the steroids down slowly and increase your anti-inflammatory drugs." All I heard was tapering steroids. I was relieved. Because of taking prednisone, a steroid, the adrenal gland turns off because it doesn't have to do what it's meant to do. When I stopped taking the prednisone, the adrenal gland didn't turn on right away, so I didn't have the benefit of its production of the steroids that my body needed, and therefore I had to taper slowly, regardless of my frustrating steroid symptoms. It had been more than six months of high-dosage steroids and not only was it wearing on me, but also my family, friends, and associates. Most of my family and friends didn't know I was on medications, they just thought I was becoming bitchy. I had snapped at everyone, including Shelly. I used every bit of discipline to keep him from knowing how really agitated and angry I felt, but sometimes steroids were more powerful than determination.

"What did the doctor say?" my sister Susan questioned, as we chatted on the phone, following my UCLA appointment. I could hear her sip her coffee while I munched on a bag of tortilla chips for a breakfast snack, trying not to make them crunch into the phone.

"Not much. They tested my adrenal gland again, and it finally kicked in, so we can start tapering the steroids," I answered, grabbing another handful of chips.

I couldn't wait to taper the steroids, because while taking such high dosages I couldn't stop eating. I couldn't stop anything. I was on a moving sidewalk that ran beneath my feet. Feet that now felt good, masked with steroids. What little pain I had was easily controlled with a pain pill. I almost convinced myself that my disease was gone, but it wasn't. RA hid under all the steroids, ready to strike with a vengeance as the steroids were withdrawn. I was trying to be positive, but would the increased anti-inflammatory drugs work?

"We're going to Hawaii for a week," my husband announced the following night as he walked in the door at his usual hour of seven o'clock. The candles were lit, Dave Koz played his smooth, sweet jazz in the background, and a Gelson's chicken potpie baked in the oven. I was determined to make up for my steroid behavior and be the good wife. "Both of us have been working too hard. I decided we need some fun, so I booked a week in Maui," Shelly beamed, proud of the good news.

I rushed into his arms. Hawaii. Lounging in a cabana for two while the tropical breezes cooled our bodies would be delicious. Romantic evenings with the shutters opened to the sound of the crashing waves. It sounded fantastic. As I held on tight to this magnificent man who had anticipated my needs, I realized I didn't have a bathing suit that fit! I had to stop eating. I must exercise more. I had two weeks to achieve some sort of improved shape and clear my calendar for a much-needed week of R & R.

Over the next two weeks my steroid-induced manic mode came in handy. I stayed on the treadmill endlessly. I drank Slim Fast in all its artificial flavors that somehow left the same chemical aftertaste in my mouth. I even ate AYDS, the popular diet-suppressant candies that tasted like chocolate or caramel, always with coffee so they would expand in my stomach. I tried to stay away from the breadbasket at dinner. It was one thing for Shelly to see me in soft candlelight, but in a bathing suit in bright sunlight?

A getaway was exactly what we needed. Recently my colleagues and friends had become suspicious. I obviously was not as good at deception as I thought I was. My lies compounded. When it came to my edgy and irritated behavior I couldn't remember what excuse I used. Several friends begin to question me.

"Is everything okay with work, Christine?"

"How are you and Shelly doing?"

"Fine, great, everything's perfect," I lied.

"You seem different, are you sure you're okay?"

"Just this crazy, busy, wonderful life. Really I'm fine," I said, and quickly changed the subject.

This was the first time friends had been vocal about the changes in my personality. No one brought up the changes in my body. The realization that people were suspicious jarred me into a desperate need to control. The two weeks before Maui became a race to get my whirling diseased life in some type of order. First, to take my weight down with more exercise and less food. Second, to conceal my weight with camouflaging clothes. Sneakers, the only shoes I could wear, had become my trademark. I had every color and style.

"I didn't realize sneakers were so in right now," one of my stylist associates mentioned, looking down at my khaki-colored, army-boot-style shoes. "You have to be very confident to wear THOSE," she glared.

"They're totally chic—where have you been?—and sooo comfy," I replied in my most elitist tone.

On the flight from LA to Maui, Shelly and I planned our week, the biggest decision being where we would eat, what books we would read, and which cabana we would reserve. My suitcase was packed with loose-fitting tent dresses, cover-up bathing suits, and a gigantic pareu that wrapped stylishly around my body to get me discreetly from the water to a lounge chair. I had managed to lose a few pounds, but only a few. The AYDS and Slim Fast tamed my appetite a bit, but the steroids offset everything, and my body demanded food. Steroids were always hungry.

Our week in Maui was perfect except for the steroids. Luckily they were working on my joints, keeping the inflammation down. While they worked on my pain, they took their inevitable toll on my mind and body. The march of the steroid army continued, even as my doctor tried to slowly decrease my dosage. I was still so jumpy and irritable. Only a steroid-driven me would find fault with the Hawaiian breezes messing up my hair. And the nights were endless, steroids making it almost impossible for me to sleep. I was sure that Shelly could sense it, but he slept like a baby— innocent and unaware. I knew it was partially my fault for keeping so much from him. How I envied and resented his peace.

Over breakfast on the hotel patio, with the ocean breezes caressing us, Shelly and I had one of our intense talks about life. It was like life as we knew it before I became sick. Not one mention of disease, work, or family issues. For an hour we slipped back into our pre-RA time, filled with vacation plans for the future, holiday celebrations, and painting a room in our home. Things we had put on the back burner for the past two years. Life when it was uncomplicated. Life as I always dreamed it would be when I lived in my childhood pretend world.

Books, television, and the few movies my mom took me to or we watched on TV together were my salvation. They offered a life I wanted to relate to while showing me that there was more to the life than what I was experiencing. They gave me the tools to create my own pretend world when I was at my boarded-out homes. In my head I was in a happy environment, living with my mom. I had a real family with a dad and brothers and sisters. It was only in my heart that the reality still lingered.

Later that day, cuddled up in our beach cabana, book in hand, I appeared to be reading but I wasn't. My mind raced, trying to figure it all out. On one hand my pain was manageable. On the other, my body was much worse. I had no control over the effects of the steroids. If I had done research I would have understood this was normal for high dosages of steroids over a long term. But I didn't. In hindsight I knew it was only because I wanted relief and didn't care about consequences. At first I had to have the drugs to get me through crisis situations. When I had to be on TV and woke up unable to walk, a few pills, and I was back on track. Then for my methotrexate lung poisoning, high dosages dripped through IVs into my arm to heal my damaged lungs. Now I needed them to compensate for my adrenal gland suppression. My dependency kept growing. The negative steroid effects kept taking over. And waiting, hiding behind the false steroid-induced sense of improvement, the RA army was gathering its own momentum. Ready to march over my body once the steroids got out of their way. The war between steroids and rheumatoid arthritis to overpower my body was in full force.

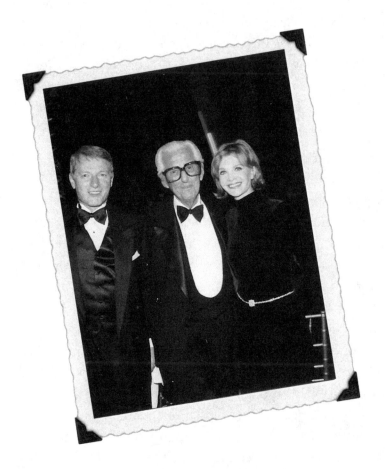

Shelly and I with the chairman of Universal Studios and the most powerful man in Hollywood, Lew Wasserman.

10

An *ET* Christmas

Christmas was one of the busiest and most exciting seasons for my work. All the shows wanted holiday segments. Fashions to wear, gifts to give, New Year's Eve makeup that glowed, resolutions for looking good for the new year. My work calendar would fill up mid-November and go right up to Christmas Eve. I always seemed to be flying home on packed planes just in time to make Christmas with my own family. And I loved it. I was past the dismal childhood Christmas holidays and into the glamour of the television holidays, where anything and everything was perfect, fantasy-like, and fun. Just my cup of tea.

Having just returned from my annual Thanksgiving "Thanks For Giving" week of makeovers with Regis and Kathie Lee, where we made over a deserving person each day, everyone from a daughter who gave a kidney to her father, to a woman who had fostered hundreds of children in her home—only unlike my childhood experiences, she adored these children and kept in touch with them. There was never a dry eye in the audience. Heartfelt holiday emotion.

My next assignment was with *Entertainment Tonight*. I loved doing this show because it was a nighttime show and always shot on location, totally different from my live, in-studio daytime programs. My producer was Bonnie Tiegel, one of the nicest people in the business. We met working on the local KTLA Morning News. Bonnie went on to produce at *ET,* I went on to national shows like *Live* and *The Today Show,* but we always kept in touch. Bonnie is the kind of person who, with all her success (she is now a senior producer for *ET* and *The Insider*), never lets go of her friends. You e-mail her, she responds immediately. No phone call is ever not returned. She praises good work and follows up every segment with a DVD of the segment and a handwritten thank-you note. This may sound like normal behavior to you, but in the television world this is unusual, very unusual. The only other notes I ever received from executives during my more than twenty-five years on TV were from Oprah. Both Bonnie's and Oprah's notes are preserved in plastic sleeves in my "favorites box." To me it says everything about the two of them as human beings.

My freelance work at *ET* consisted of special assignments. I would come up with a theme, and Bonnie would tweak it to the show's audience and give it the green light. This holiday assignment was about where celebrities do their holiday shopping. My prep work included scouting out locations and talking with store owners about what celebrities frequented their stores. Since it was early December, most celebrities hadn't shopped yet, but once I located their favorite stores, I could show the things the owners felt they might buy, some things they had already bought, or things that I thought fit in with their personalities or the person they were dating or married to. The result was a fun, interesting, celebrity-filled segment. Perfect for *Entertainment Tonight,* or as it's referred to in the business, *ET.*

It takes at least one day of shooting, sometimes more, to put together a three- to five-minute piece for the show. I was assigned a director, a cameraman, and a soundman.

We were given a call date and time and met at the first location, often meeting each other for the first time. The level of crew and talent at *ET* was always the best, so no one had to prove themselves. It was a given—if you were on *ET*, you knew what you were doing. At each location they set up lighting, always caring about the way talent looked. After doing many news segments where a camera is pointed in your face with one glaring bright light attached to the top, having someone adjust lights and do camera checks to see how I looked was a treat. News is not concerned with how you look—they want the story. *ET* wants glamour, and they spend the time and money to create it.

My first location was Lisa Kline's boutique on Robertson Boulevard, one of the most popular and unique shopping streets in Los Angeles. Lisa had a big reputation for celebrity clients, both men and women. Her women's boutique was on one side of the street, the men's directly across the street. We started in the women's store, where whimsical flannel pajamas were all the rage with celebrities; think the antithesis of Victoria's Secret. Covered in cartoon characters, clouds, or white fluffy sheep, boutiques couldn't keep the pajamas on the shelves. Standing behind a table covered in these fun PJ's, I talked into the camera—as if it were my best friend—telling them how Reese Witherspoon was planning on giving these as holiday gifts to many of her girlfriends. The camera zoomed in on the colorful designs and then moved in tight to my face for a close-up. Luckily I was not in one of my moon-shaped-face periods and looking more like my normal self, so I was able to smile and play into the camera. Take No.1 complete.

We crossed the store for Take No.2, designer T-shirts for men. The common T-shirt had recently taken on a new look, made of expensive fabrics with a prestigious designer label inside. Instead of white T-shirts in a three-pack for ten dollars, purchases could now run up in the hundreds of dollars, and celebrities were buying them up. "What better gift if Tom Cruise or Richard Gere were on your shopping list?" I asked the camera, holding up the new, slim-cut, high V-neck T-shirts. What man wouldn't look like a star in a two-hundred dollar Armani T-shirt?

We then moved over to the chichi stretch on Sunset Boulevard known as Sunset Plaza. It is a collection of outdoor cafes and boutiques where celebrities love to shop and eat. First stop was the popular Billy Martin's, which sells high-end Western wear. A pair of alligator boots topping the price scale of well over $1,500 were my suggestion as the perfect gift for Arnold Schwarzenegger to give his wife, Maria Shriver. I never saw her wearing them at the private beach club they belong to, but then who wears Western boots at the beach? I'm positive Arnold took my suggestion.

The hot new bath shop Waterworks had just opened on the Sunset Plaza, featuring everything from designer tubs to luxurious bathrobes. I had planned ahead and brought along a replica of Kobe Bryant's Laker jersey to place under one of their robes. Untying the thick white robe, I revealed the jersey to the camera, telling what a nice combination it would be under Kobe's Christmas tree. The director loved it, and had me do several close-ups of removing the tie on the robe for the reveal. Luckily my meds were working, and my hands weren't swollen and red. Even my feet, although outfitted in some cool-looking sneakers that the camera didn't catch, were cooperating. I was having one of my better days, and I was so appreciative.

Our last stop was Neil Lane, one of the most talented and desired jewelers in town. His jewels adorned the necks of some of Hollywood's biggest stars at the awards shows. Celebrities clamored to wear his diamonds on the red carpet. His engagement rings were every woman's dream. Jason Patric was dating Julia Roberts after he actually stole her right from under her fiancé Kiefer Sutherland's nose. So who better to recommend buying a Neil Lane holiday diamond for than Jason for Julia? I know it seemed a bit rushed, but in Hollywood engagements are made and broken in hours. The director smiled, knowing the audience would love it. A little insider gossip, for the queen of gossip shows.

After a few bridges, where I walk down the street toward the camera, or move in and out of stores as I'm talking, we wrapped in the late afternoon. Bridges are used by the editors to move from one place to another. By now I was experienced and could walk and talk at the same time. But I remember when I first did bridges for KABC Eyewitness News in Los Angeles as their fashion reporter. I was new and totally green and it would take many takes to get one good walking/talking bridge. There's something about putting one foot in front of the other while trying to "sparkle" in front of a camera moving backward in front of you that takes time to adjust to. It's anything but natural in person, but on the screen it looks as if you're taking the viewer shopping with you. Then we shot some more close-ups of gift ideas, long shots of storefronts, and casual shots of shoppers at work.

Now the segment was out of my hands. The director took the tapes to the studio, and the editor took over. The following week, there I was on *ET* with dancing Christmas trees and shiny ornaments on the screen while the talent introduced my segment. They added cash registers with the over-the-top prices. Nobody edits and puts a segment together like *ET.* It was perfect for the holidays. Because it has a huge viewing audience, *ET* always made my phone ring with compliments. And then came the lovely note from Bonnie. A television Christmas doesn't get any better.

11

Stable Until Ready

My life, three years after my diagnosis, was now totally defined by my chronic rheumatoid arthritis. My secret was still safe even though my health was not. Over the last year I had been on Azulfidine, Imuran, Plaquenil, Epogen shots for anemia, and Cytoxan, gold Shots, and of course lots of Zantac to coat my stomach for the drug onslaught. After reading the information on Cytoxan, a drug used in cancer chemotherapy, I stopped reading. It was too depressing to learn all the side effects when I didn't have a choice. Without medication I wouldn't be able to walk. Still Dr. Kalunian kept holding out hope.

"There's some really good drugs in testing programs, we just need to keep you stable until they're ready," he told me. Stable was something I couldn't relate to. Up to now he would start me on a new combination of drugs and even if they helped my RA, it was only a matter of time before my lab work came back with issues. We had to constantly change medications because my system wouldn't tolerate the side effects. Or my hair started falling out in tufts, or my hearing was affected. It was always something.

"Christine, I think you need to get your hearing checked. I've noticed that you don't seem to hear a lot of what I say,"

Shelly said to me one morning as he called me to the phone and I didn't respond. "It seems to be getting worse."

I barely noticed. I was consumed with medications and doctors' appointments. My work schedule now revolved around my time at UCLA. My social life revolved around my medical life. I felt like a revolving door running in circles out of control.

I also felt like a supersleuth, always padding the lies. If I slipped and let anyone know the state of my health my career could be in jeopardy. Television was a small world.

"Sorry, I can't join you for lunch. I have a meeting with my literary agent," I lied to my girlfriends.

"I hate to cancel at the last minute but Shelly and I have to go out of town," I said to our couple friends so I could cancel dinner plans that my queasy, overmedicated stomach wouldn't allow me to attend.

I had come up with other excuses at work. "Just going to pick up a few things," I told my New York assistants as I rushed into a doctor's office at Eighty-ninth and Park for the weekly gold Shots Dr. Kalunian had arranged for me to get when I was in New York. Travel didn't matter, the continuity of the medicine was mandatory. I'd run into the doctor's office, climb up on the exam table, and lay on my stomach as they pumped what was called gold into my tush. It might have been gold, but it was thick and it hurt as it was plunged in with a big needle, and no, I didn't turn a golden bronze tan color, nor set the security alarms off at the airports. Gold Shots had been around for years and so far they weren't doing much for my RA. I decided I'd rather have my gold in a pair of hoop earrings or a new charm for my bracelet. Today gold has been replaced by newer treatments with superior benefits and less risk. It's considered an old treatment that is hardly used now, but a few patients were put in remission with gold, and although it's harder to obtain, they still have the injections.

"Trying to grow out my bangs," I answered when asked about my latest hairpiece to cover up my thinning hair from the toxic Cytoxan medication. My desk had a stack of blue lined note cards that I used on television segments to keep all of the designer and store names organized. The blue color was for TV because it wasn't as noticeable as white on camera. I was beginning to feel I needed blue note cards to juggle the various lies I told friends and colleagues. Would my cover be blown if I overlapped my stories?

I was good at fabricating the truth. My childhood fantasies enabled me to escape my foster-home sadness. Now that same daydream world worked for me almost to the point of believing I didn't have a disease until the pain brought me back to reality. My childhood didn't prepare me for the lies and deceits I now needed to keep my secret. I asked myself what choice I had. I had worked my entire life to get where I was, and now my own body was fighting to take it all away. The career in television that made me feel needed and successful, the marriage that made me feel as complete as I was capable of and more loved than I had ever experienced. The exciting lifestyle that once was only in my imagination and now was in my daily schedule. I couldn't let it all go. I had to fight to hold on. With each day, week, month, and year the fight became more complicated.

"I would normally love to do that segment, but I'm booked to work in LA," I lied when I knew I couldn't add anything else to my workload. My days of running from one job to another, from meeting to meeting, and always being able to squeeze in something else were finished. I now had to monitor my days and my evenings. With Shelly's social commitments a necessity, I had to cut mine way back. Most of my days now consisted of medical appointments, a little work, resting, and medicating so I could get through the evening's obligations.

By the end of the month Dr. Kalunian prescribed Epogen shots for the anemia that sapped my energy. The good news was that I was now off the prednisone. The bad news was that the hyped-up steroid energy disappeared with the drug. In only a few weeks we learned the Epogen shots would not give me the boost we hoped. I was exhausted most of the time, and now my camouflaging pain pills seemed to wear off earlier and earlier during the social evenings.

I needed a second opinion. I needed something, anything, to help. Dr. Wallace was the chief of rheumatology at Cedars-Sinai. His reputation in the medical community was stellar. Dr. Kalunian recommended him and understood why I needed another opinion. I couldn't get my head around Dr. Kalunian's hope for drugs that were currently only in research. I had lost my patience waiting. I needed to deal better with the moment. I needed to keep up with my husband. How much longer would he sit home watching TV with me when we were supposed to be at a political fund-raiser? How many excuses could we get away with for leaving events early because my pain was too intense to sit any longer with a smile on my face? I felt threatened emotionally and physically.

On a beautiful spring day in early March, I walked into the Beverly Hills Medical Clinic on Beverly Boulevard. I felt optimistic for the first time in ages. There had to be something that could work. The office waiting room was filled with older people. I recognized the ravages of RA on their bodies. Some had distorted hands. Others wore orthopedic shoes. One woman walked with a cane, another man with a walker. The room's decor matched. The walls were a drab beige. The lined-up chairs were worn and tired. The magazines all outdated. Not a single window allowed the spring day inside.

Dr. Wallace's nurse handed me a form to list the drugs I had taken. I used small print that extended into the margins in order to fit them all in. "Thanks, Dr. Wallace will be with you shortly," the nurse behind the frosted glass window said, a lie told so well she could easily get a job in entertainment. Based on the number of people in the waiting room, I knew it would not be shortly.

Dr. Wallace was not a man who smiled. When he entered a room he sucked any possibility of lightness right out of it. His face was set in a down-turned, sad expression when he greeted me. It didn't bode well for someone in desperate search of hope.

"Well, Christine, seems like you've tried a lot of medications," he said, looking over my newly filled-out chart. After checking my tender, inflamed joints, he sat down on the swivel stool and continued to stare at my chart as if waiting for answers to pop out at him. "I think we should try to rechallenge you with low doses of methotrexate. Just because you had a reaction to it once doesn't mean you will again," he finally said, looking me sternly in the eyes.

Rechallange me? METHOTREXATE? The drug that put me in the hospital for more than a week and almost killed me? The drug that forced me to take steroids for a year just to clear up my lungs? Was he kidding? My body had been challenged enough trying to survive the side effects of methotrexate.

Trying to keep my voice from screeching, I answered, "I really don't want to go on methotrexate again after my last experience."

"Well, you only have a few choices," he said as he peered over his smudged half glasses, giving me the "so you choose to disagree with the doctor" tone of voice. "There's some experimental work being done in San Francisco where they drain your blood, clean it, and then replace it. Not much data, but you might want to check it out."

Drain my blood and clean it? I thought I read about that being done once to heroin addicts. It sounded like some weird vampire carnival game.

"Then there's the new TNF-alpha drug they're testing in London," he continued, never missing a beat, now looking at my chart so he didn't have to look at me. "If I were you I would beg, borrow, or steal to try to get in one of the testing programs in London. These drugs are a totally new approach to immune diseases. They actually block the body's system from attacking itself."

"How would I even begin?" I asked, the sophisticated city of London sounding far better than draining my blood in San Francisco.

"I really can't advise you. The drug is manufactured by a company called Immunex, and I think they're headquartered in Seattle. That's about all I know except for the testing in London. Depending on how the tests in London go, they could be in the United States in a few years."

I didn't think my emotional state had a few years. I doubted that my career could hold up a few more years, and my marriage? Would my husband finally realize that he didn't get what he bargained for?

I guess, in hindsight, my mom didn't get what she bargained for, either. She lost her mom at eight and when her dad remarried quickly, she and my aunt were really not very welcome in the new household. An aunt took them in for a while, but basically the twins were on their own at fifteen, moving from Arkansas to California, where jobs for beautiful young girls were touted. My aunt, being the stronger one, was my mom's only mother figure.

And then my dad, the handsome policeman who swept my eighteen-year-old mother off her feet and got her pregnant, turned out to not be the man she fell in love with. Now with him out of the picture, she was once again on her own with my aunt, only now they had me, a needy, confused little girl. When I asked her one day where my daddy was, because I really didn't remember him before he went away, she replied with another question: "What made you ask that, Chrissie?" I guess I told her all the kids at school had daddies and I wanted one too, or something that a five-year-old would say. My mom's reply was to ask me if I wanted to go to Clifton's Cafeteria for dinner, my favorite. It took my mind off of my question, thinking of the flag with the red tip that would be in my food, enabling me to visit the treasure chest of gifts. Looking back, this might have been my first experience with the denial that would become such an important part of my life both as a child and as a chronically ill adult.

Dr. Wallace's voice brought me back to reality. "Sorry I can't be more help. There are still other combinations of the drugs you have been on that we can try. I'll call Dr. Kalunian and talk with him about some alternatives." And he stood and walked out the door, leaving me more frustrated than before.

That evening, Shelly and I walked around the corner from our condo to our favorite Chinese restaurant, Xi'an on Canon, for a relaxed dinner. No black ties, no business meetings, just the two of us at a small table by the window with delicious tofu and chicken in black bean sauce and healthy brown rice.

"Looks like the Kitty Kelley talk show is not going to go," Shelly told me, trying to hide his frustration by mixing the apricot sauce with the hot mustard. "We sold it in all the major markets until the word came from upstairs that it was over. No official reason was given." The Wassermans and the Reagans were good friends so the speculation was that Reagan might have put in a call to Wasserman and killed the show. Some people felt that Reagan never got over the book Kelley wrote on Nancy, saying she had an affair with Sinatra.

I knew how disappointed he was because of the hours and money that went into a pilot that created great buzz in the industry. Kitty Kelley, the best-selling author, was even better on camera than in print.

"Christine, are you listening?" Shelly's sharp tone woke me out of my daydreaming.

"Sorry, I was thinking of the treatment alternatives Dr. Wallace gave me today."

"Can't we talk about something else besides your health while we're eating?" Shelly responded with a new edge I hadn't heard in his voice before.

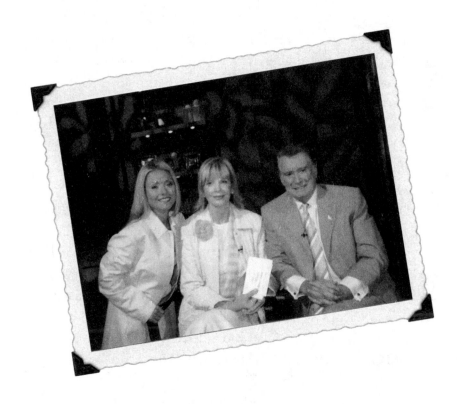

My twenty-five year association with Regis continued with the delightful Kelly Ripa.

12

Here Today, Gone Tomorrow

JANUARY, 1994

In my business I am always looking at what's next. A new, different show to add to my list of shows. For me it's two reasons. First, I need to always feel I am growing and improving—it's the "need for approval" gene from my childhood. Second, I know how vulnerable television is. A new producer takes over (and this happens all the time—as a show's ratings fall you can count the days until the executive producer will be replaced) and you can be out of a job as the new producer brings in all his own talent. Cleaning house; it happens in most businesses.

Currently I am a regular on *Live,* which is a great gig. I do some special assignments for *Entertainment Tonight,* which is exciting and different. I have done three *Oprah* shows, which is the brass ring. I do Fox Network News on most of my visits to New York, which is quick, easy, newsy; no models, fewer props, an in-and-out gig. And then sometimes, especially around the holidays, I will add a New York or Los Angeles local morning show for a gift segment, accessory segment, or tabletop segment. A tabletop segment is where you make a display and go down the table showing the best shoes, bags, or gift items for the season. Sometimes the phone will ring with something different and unique on a network show that is a nice change of pace, and sometimes you have to pitch and plan and make something new happen for yourself. One of my long-term goals had always been to be a regular on *The Today Show.* It's more of a major news, reported-segment type of show. The show wouldn't conflict with my work on *Live.* Michael, *Live's* executive producer, is very possessive of his talents and doesn't want them appearing on any show that is on any station at the same time as his, which makes it hard on the talents, because *Live* is a syndicated show, meaning that it's on different stations at different times across the country. This is a deal breaker with Michael, and so those of us who worked at *Live,* even without written contracts, played by the rules. When I checked with Michael, he said he didn't have any problem with me adding *Today* to my freelance list because the shows were not in competition with each other. Permission granted, now it was up to me to set my sights and go to work on the television dating game, because in many ways it is like pursuing a date with someone you have been dreaming about for a long time. It takes patience and persistence. And even with my arthritis moving in and out of my body on a whim based on medicines either working or not working, I liked the chase. I liked the dating game. I may have arthritis, but my determination not to let arthritis rule my life still remained strong, at least on most days.

For *The Today Show,* the dating game began and ended with the executive producer, Steve Friedman. Steve of course knew who I was. Everyone in daytime television knows about everyone who works in daytime television—it's a small world when it comes to players. I had been on *The Today Show* several times with my first book, *Quickstyle,* and I was captivated by the energy at *Today.* The early morning mood in their studios vibrated with electricity. As I set up my tabletop display, this time on shoes, along with their talented set designer, music blared from a rehearsing band and everyone in the studio, even though in a sleepy haze of the dark morning, would find their feet tapping to the beat as they went about their work. *The Today Show* was used to being number one in the early hours, and the daily pressure of remaining there made everyone work at the top of his or her game. They had been pleased with my previous segments, but now I wanted to try for a regular gig. I loved the high-stakes television *The Today Show* played.

Now I had to pursue Steve Friedman. I met him on the set the first time I did the show and kept in touch. He knew I was ambitious and wanted to do more on his show, and he didn't say no, it just took him a long time to say yes. Steve is an interesting character. Meeting in his office is like a test. He talked to you while corresponding on the computer, taking phone calls, and swinging his beloved Chicago Cubs baseball bat. It's almost as if he was trying to see if you could keep your pitch focus while he obviously ignored you, letting you know that on his priority list you were not even close to the top. In hindsight I think his goal was to see how much you wanted to be on the show. How deep your passion was. He often made people feel like they were in the way, making it even harder to stay focused and motivated unless you were totally passionate. And I was.

It took ten calls to get through to him, and when you did he wanted to know in twenty seconds—if you were lucky enough to get that much time—why you were taking his time. I wanted an appointment. I wanted to pitch him. I wanted to be a regular on his show. I knew I was right for the show and I think he did as well, but he wanted to see how badly I wanted it and to some crazy extent, I enjoyed playing his game. After many, many calls to his patient and friendly assistant Tami, Steve finally got on the phone.

"You really like it there at *Live with Regis and Kathie Lee*?" he asked, baiting me.

"I love it, but I want to do more extensive stories, more fashion reporting."

"And Gelman's okay with you being on our show?"

"He's fine, our agreement is I can do any show that is not on opposite him, and because *Live* is syndicated, that's not always easy, but you're on earlier. He actually likes the idea," I pitched. You had to talk fast and to the point with Steve; he didn't have time for chitchat.

"So, what do you want from me?" he asked me in his gruff, you're-bothering-me voice.

"I want to be a correspondent on your show. I have an idea to do segments where I make house calls on people needing style advice. I go in, address their problems, and fix them, like a style doctor." I talked quickly before he got lost in his computer. Steve has a short attention span, but I had his attention. I wondered if some other talent was sitting in his office being ignored while he talked to me.

"Example?"

"A young couple with small children both work. Their mornings are hectic and disorganized. I go in and organize them, everything from setting up the coffee the night before to cleaning out closets and putting outfits together a week ahead," I said, thinking I could hear his mind clicking.

"We need to do a screen test with you and the talent. Give me a list of ideas, make some about fashion trends," and the phone clicked. Steve had just hung up on me, but it didn't matter, I was ecstatic, I had an assignment.

The next day, sitting at my desk with swollen, puffy fingers that ached as I pressed on the computer keys, I put my list together and sent it to Steve. Arthritis flares when it wants to, sometimes for no apparent reason. It doesn't care if you are in the dating game or not. It doesn't care if you need your fingers to type or your feet to walk; arthritis does exactly what it wants, and if you want a life you have to adapt as best you can. So, one finger at a time, I painfully typed ten strong fashion/style segments. I was just glad I was in the privacy of my condo and not in public view.

After another dozen phone calls during which Tami said he was in a meeting, he was out of the office, or could I call him back tomorrow, he finally, through Tami, approved the story on long johns as outerwear, a new trend that was just hitting the New York runways that was not on my list, but rather in some magazine Steve was looking at them while talking to me on the phone.

"I'm assigning you a young, talented producer in the LA office, Audrey Kolina. She will call you and set up the shoot," Steve said when he finally took my call. Most people would have given up. Steve can be gruff, but under that stern exterior is a teddy bear. He always left me with just enough hope to keep me pursuing. By the time he gave me the assignment he knew I was serious, I wanted the job, and he was willing to give me a try.

Because the trend was so new, all I could locate on it was runway footage and the article Steve had read. I needed more. After researching I found that Seattle was the town where the trend had started. I shared this information with Audrey, who I had only met by phone so far, and she replied, "Then we're going to Seattle."

The following week, Audrey, a soundman, a cameraman, and I were on the plane. I had located a *Northern Exposure* type of bar where the locals were starting to wear thermal tops or thermal pants mixed in with their traditional flannels and denim. We had permission to shoot. I sat next to Audrey on the plane. For whatever reason we clicked right off the bat, or at least I did. And she, being a reporter, asked me a lot of questions. By the time we landed she knew most of the details of my life. And I'm sure the cameraman and soundman in back of me heard, too. What had I done? I was always so good at keeping my personal and professional life separate. Somehow Audrey's easy manner made me a motormouth, and I went to sleep in the Seattle hotel that night wondering why did she need the details of my divorce, or really, why did I feel free enough to tell her? The only thing about my life I didn't tell her was my arthritis, thank goodness. What had she done to open the floodgates when I was usually so guarded? And with a major producer at *The Today Show*? I couldn't sleep for fear of the consequences my soap opera tirade might cause.

The bar turned out to be perfect, filled with young, hip Northwesterners. The only problem was Seattle—usually so rainy and cool—was having a heat wave in January and nobody was wearing thermals. Strapless corseted tops, cut-off T-shirts, and bra tops looked more like Hollywood than Seattle. The guys were in short-sleeve plaid shirts and sleeveless T-shirts, not a thermal in sight. In the crowded bar, with our lights blazing, we got interviews about the trend, but we had to shoot above the neck. "Don't worry, we can lay runway footage over their voices," Audrey said in her calm, take-control manner. And I worried again that Audrey knew too much. The only thing I had left out of my life was my RA, and had the flight been longer I wondered if I would have even revealed that. Had Audrey been a therapist before she worked in television?

The crowded bar was hot and sweaty, Seattle not being big on air conditioning. Between the camera lights and the dancing bodies there was very little air in the room. I was becoming overheated and light-headed. "Just need some fresh air," I said to Audrey, heading toward the door. "Wait, I'll come with you," Audrey said, pushing through the crowds. "What a scene, but I think we got some good footage," Audrey said, watching me lean against the stucco building. "Christine, are you okay? You look pale."

"Fine, I'm fine, just needed to get out of the crowd," I lied. Tonight, even my stylish sneakers weren't comfortable.

Back at NBC Burbank studios Audrey and I put the piece together. Between the bar, the runway, and some department-store footage of thermals, I had a story. Tami, Steve's assistant, called to say the audition segment was scheduled for the following week. I would tape it with Bryant Gumbel right after the regular show.

There is an energy in the early hours of the morning at *The Today Show* that is infectious. Most days there is a band or singer practicing, so the stages are filled with music. The lights from the studio are so bright against the early morning darkness. It's such a contrast. The streets around the studio are dark and quiet, but when you step inside the big black doors in Rockefeller Center, it's like the middle of the day, a beehive of activity. Nobody is looking tired and sleepy. They are moving fast, thinking fast, and into their work. Even though my segment would be taped after the nine o'clock hour finished, I had to arrive early for hair and makeup and to be ready to go onstage the minute the show was over and Bryant was ready. You don't keep talent waiting.

I wore my favorite skirted suit. I wore nylons with my sneakers, my heels packed in my tote for the last-minute change. I had iced my red and swollen feet that morning, praying that they would squeeze into my heels. A fashion reporter can't wear sneakers on *The Today Show*. I gulped one pain pill before I left my hotel, a bottle of chocolate milk to coat my stomach, and had another pain pill tucked into my suit jacket pocket, just in case. I didn't sleep well because I was excited. My future with *The Today Show* rested on this audition. I had to be great. Adding to the pressure, I had heard that Bryant can be tough if he doesn't think you're up to speed.

The stage manager placed me in a club chair with an empty matching one across from me. Pictures of winter trees were hanging in back. My feet were bulging out of my shoes so I tried to place them crossed in a position to hide as much as possible. I gulped the second pain pill, gathering saliva in my mouth rather than asking for water and having someone see me.

And then Bryant walked on the set. So far I had only seen him on TV. That morning Jane Pauley walked by me with her hair wrapped in a towel, freshly washed. Even in a towel she was impressive with a welcoming smile. But Bryant was more serious. He walked on, sat in the seat across from me, and leaned forward with his hand out. "Hi, I'm Bryant." I put my hand out, trying to hold it steady, hoping he wouldn't shake it too hard and start the throbbing pain that had dulled somewhat after my second pain pill. "Hi, I'm Christine Kunzelman." He nodded and looked down at his notes. I had always been impressed by Bryant on television. He is smart, quick, and to the point in an interview. What I wasn't prepared for was how handsome he was in person. When he looks you in the eyes, he looks you in the eyes. The kind of look that you feel in the pit of your stomach.

"Really, long johns in public?" he asked me, a half smile on his face as if to say, "are you kidding?"

"They're the hottest thing on the fashion runways. Underwear has been making itself more obvious for a while now, but this type of underwear is practical, it's also comfortable, and, mixed with other items, now fashionable," I tried to convince him.

"Okay, let's roll," he said, as if to say, show me, I'm not so sure.

He introduced me and went right into the question, "So Christine, you think people are really going to wear long johns to dinner?" And I jumped on the bandwagon and did my thing. Five minutes and one taped piece later, Bryant stood, offered his hand again, and said, "Nice job." I stayed in my club chair, knowing between my feet and my knees that to get up quickly could put me on the floor, in front of Bryant Gumbel and the crew of *The Today Show.* And so I sat and shook his hand and said, "Thanks."

Steve called me a few days later and said you have a job. "We'll start with the hectic morning family. We're designing a logo for you. Your segments will be called 'House Calls.'" I was over the moon. But Steve's voice also implied, "Don't let me down." And Shelly's voice was filled with worry.

"Why, Christine? Why don't you slow down instead of accelerate your work schedule? You need to rest more, not work more. I don't know why you feel you have to do this."

But I knew why. Because I was still looking for that approval I didn't get as a child. That acceptance I missed in elementary schools because I moved around so much. I wanted to live in the big houses with the big players, not the "boarded-out" houses in which I spent my early years. I couldn't stop. And now, with arthritis chasing me around, trying, in my mind, to take me down, I couldn't, wouldn't let it win.

Audrey and I taped the first House Calls piece at one of my friend's homes. She had an eighteen-month-old and a new baby, she had a full-time executive job at IBM, and her husband was an architect. Needless to say, their life was out of control, especially in the mornings trying to get to work in time. I bought a coffeepot that had a timer they could set to go off before they woke, cleaned out their drawers and organized their closets, putting together outfits for her with all the accessories in plastic bags,= tied around the hanger necks. I organized the children's clothes so it was easy to locate what you needed even with sleep in your eyes. No more early morning decisions to make. On tape I showed them how to be efficient, practical, and stylish. They were so elated to have some solutions—their smiles lit up on camera. I had chosen the perfect appreciative couple.

Audrey and I sat in on editing. The editor added great music, with some scenes speeded up and a clock ticking in the upper screen corner. It was perfect. The logo NBC designed for me was a house with a hair dryer, makeup brushes, and articles of clothing dancing around it. Professionally I was on cloud nine. But physically I was living on chocolate milk, trying to coat my stomach from both the food and the medication. One or the other was always making me feel nauseous.

At *The Today Show* things were going well. Steve seemed pleased, but still let me know I was in the "prove it to me" stage.

By the third segment I was organizing a single man's closet. His answer to fashion was to only wear black and white. We took the cameras into his closet, interviewed him, and then I took him shopping and added color and style to his wardrobe. "This is my favorite segment so far," Audrey complimented me as I did the voice-over for the piece. I wasn't so sure. I had been so sick that I felt I could have given more, done another interview, added something else, but my energy level was at an all-time low. I was pushing to get anything done and my stomach was not cooperating. I was barely making it through the days. Dr. Kalunian was once again changing my meds, trying to find some balance, but so far, my stomach was not liking anything.

"Steve Friedman is out," Audrey told me the day after we finished putting the men's style piece together. "Michael Bass, his number two, is taking over. I'm sending the piece to him today, so you'll probably be on air next week."

Steve Friedman out? Steve Friedman was a giant in morning television. I couldn't believe what I was hearing. It didn't dawn on me then that this could impact me, I was too concentrated on trying to control my disease and my career.

But next week came and went and no air date. And then the call came.

"Christine, Michael doesn't like the piece. Said he didn't learn anything new from it," Audrey told me. I sat back in my chair, shocked. I thought it was loaded with good fashion tips. "Let's just let this play out. There is a lot of upheaval around here with Steve gone, once things settle down we can talk to Michael and see what he wants to do. It's a good piece, don't worry."

Over the next few weeks I didn't hear anything. I had never met Michael Bass. I was one of Steve's people, one of his very new people. I knew that couldn't be a good thing with Steve gone. Television is interesting, like most big businesses. Talent is often associated with the team who discovers them, or hires them. When a new team captain comes into play, they often like to clean house, especially with part-time talent or lower-end executives. They want to put their own stamp on things. The stamp that says, "This is my team, I am the captain."

I tried to get in touch with Michael, thinking if I could talk to him, meet him in person, everything would be okay. But he didn't respond.

"Just give it some time," Audrey counseled me. I knew Audrey was on my side, but she was also pregnant with her second child, her little boy Jay barely two years old. Audrey had her hands full reporting on late-breaking news stories and dealing with other reporter talents covering hard news. Fashion was something Steve Friedman had assigned her because she was good and also in Los Angeles. The healthy me would have fought tooth and nail. Called and re-called. I wouldn't have sat silently at home, drinking my chocolate milk. But this was a new me—a frustrated, overmedicated me, trying to balance it all, and my inner fire was coated in so much chocolate milk, I couldn't ignite it. And so I let it disappear. Did I have any other options? Yes, I was hired, I had a logo, I was introduced as a Contributing Editor, I could have made new lists of segment ideas specifically for Michael. I could have worked my way through his assistant like I did with Tami and just assumed all was well and moved forward. I could have hounded Audrey. But a chronic disease is a roller coaster ride. Sometimes you're at the top and sometimes you're at the bottom. I was at the bottom, I couldn't get my disease under control, it was running me and not in a good direction. The show I had worked so hard to get was slipping away and all I could do was watch. I was not the Christine Kunzelman who shook Bryant's hand and played the "I won't give up" dating game with Steve Friedman. I was Christine Kunzelman with RA. I didn't like her at all, but at the time I didn't have the strength or wherewithal to change her.

It was a lot like my childhood. My mom tried to convince me not to cry when she took me back to my foster home. I would promise her I wouldn't and work hard to keep the tears back. I never wanted to hurt my mom, all I wanted was to be with her. Then the good-bye kiss would come, and she would brush her hands through my hair as if to fix it one last time and then quickly walk away, never looking back. And the tears would start rolling down my cheeks. Silent, angry, frustrated tears. The sadness had taken over, and regardless of how much I wanted to please my mom, the sadness always won. And so I cried because my life was so out of control and there was nothing I could do to change it.

And so *The Today Show* was gone. It had taken so long to make it, and then it was over and for the first time in my life I gave up too easily. Could I have made a difference if I fought to hold on? I didn't know. All I knew was that arthritis had taken it away, or so it seemed to me at the time. Arthritis was winning. I knew I had to get my fight back. But I couldn't, not today. Would I be my healthy, aggressive self tomorrow, next month, next year? Would I ever be me again? And just as with any ended relationship, my heart was broken, only this time my body felt broken, too.

13

Oprah, My Best Friend for a Day

The next two years were filled with more of the same. The ups and downs of rheumatoid arthritis and the ups and downs of television. Nothing too extreme, just living from day to day and doing the best I could. And then, out of the blue, a call comes that takes away all the pain of arthritis and the disappointments of television. In this case it was a call from Oprah.

I was in the dressing room at the WABC-TV studios in New York having just finished shooting *Live*. My assistant Amy pushed through the crowded room, trying to maneuver me out the door.

"You've got to get out of here. You'll miss your plane," Amy pleaded. She always watched my back, trying to protect me from the craziness at the studios where we taped *Live with Regis and Kathie Lee*. In our four-by-five dressing room there was my producer, today's completed makeover with her husband, the makeover for tomorrow's show and her daughter, my two assistants, a hairdresser, and makeup artist. There was no space and no air in the room. You would think from the frenetic atmosphere in the dressing room that I was dealing with world issues, but in reality it was only a week of Mother's Day makeovers for the show.

I had just finished my second makeover for the week. Now I needed to get to Chicago as fast as possible.

"Please, everyone, Christine has to leave NOW. Everything's under control. We'll be in constant contact with her during the day," Amy shouted over the turmoil, as she moved over to the closet to grab my coat. Pulling at my arm, Amy ushered me out through the studio's revolving front doors onto Columbus Avenue.

The town car waited to whisk me to JFK for my flight to Chicago to tape *Oprah*. "Good morning Ms. Kunzelman. I'm Danny, your driver. We're off to JFK, American Airlines, domestic, right?"

"Right," I replied, relaxing my aching body into the rich leather seats, sipping the cup of coffee Amy handed me.

I had now been living with rheumatoid arthritis for six years. Six years of introducing new drugs, mixing combinations of old drugs, and running into dead ends on all fronts. My pain was chronic. I was tired. I was depressed. I struggled daily to hold on to my career and keep my marriage as normal as possible. My survival training in foster homes turned out to be the foundation for the strength I needed during this time. My ability to live in a fantasy world came in handy. My real life was a fantasy. On paper it looked perfect. Rheumatoid arthritis had robbed me of many things, but I refused to let it ruin my life and so I forged ahead, in my stylish signature sneakers. Denial worked for me. If I looked good and acted normal, I could almost convince myself I was. With the help of pain pills, a doctor who understood my need for normalcy, and an exciting career and marriage, some days I almost was normal. On the others, the really bad days, I kept my pain to myself. I concentrated on what was good in my life, and that list was long. In the negative column it was only one issue, my health. I refused to let them merge.

Today was going to be one of my good days. There were no more great days, but I was going to be on *Oprah* so it had to be at least a good day. I sat back and savored the anticipation in the stillness and silence as we drove to the airport. I had been working since five o'clock A.M. The stress of the day had already demanded two pain pills just to cope with my inflamed joints, and at ten thirty my day was only beginning.

The first call had come weeks before as I stood in line at the pharmacy filling my prescriptions for my upcoming trip to New York.

"Christine, it's Megan Simpson, producer at *Oprah*. We have a segment next Tuesday on appropriate dressing for women. There will be three experts and we'd like you to be one." The minute I heard the word "Oprah" my heart raced. In television there was no better call. Then I thought of my bags packed at home ready for New York and ten days of television work.

My mind went into overdrive. How could I make this work? I would be in the middle of the Mother's Day makeover week on *Live with Regis and Kathie Lee,* where there was no free time. But nobody said no to Oprah. I had to make it work. I would get everything in place, and Amy could take over. Amy would need an assistant. I'd consult by phone. Amy knew the procedure. It wasn't like I was leaving her on her own. I would see the makeover in the morning, do the consultation, and figure out the direction we needed to go. It all depended on convincing the people at *Live* and *Oprah* that I could handle both. My excitement eliminated any doubt in my mind; I could do this.

"We'll bring you in on Monday, the segment is Tuesday, and you can fly back to LA that night. We'll book you at the Omni Berkshire, same as last time," the producer informed me, totally unaware of my scheduling dilemma.

I swallowed hard before I answered, every inch of my body filled with excitement. When people in line overheard the word "Oprah," every one of them was glued. This drugstore was after all Hollywood adjacent.

"Great topic for a segment, and I would love to do it. I'll actually be working close by on *Regis and Kathie Lee.*"

Silence. Was she still on the line?

"So does that mean you'll be available only when their show is over?" she asked. I could hear the change in her tone. She was probably on overload and didn't need any more complications.

"Yes, the show goes off the air at ten o'clock A.M, and I can be free for the rest of the day." I was glad the producers of *Live* couldn't hear this conversation. They depended on me to manage the makeovers during the day and deliver a completed, perfect specimen the next morning. They didn't need complications either.

"We start taping at noon, but we're taping two shows that day, so let me check and see if we can do this show second and make the times work. I'll get back to you." And she was gone.

I immediately began second-guessing myself. Did I respond correctly? Did I let her know how much I wanted to do the show? Will *Live* go crazy when they find out I might be gone the entire day when I was committed to them for the week? Will she even call back? As my mind raced, questioning my every word, the phone rang.

"Christine, Meg here. I talked to my supervising producer, and she said we're cutting it close, but we can make it work. We'll go over the segment later." Again she was gone. She didn't ask if that was okay. She worked for Oprah. She didn't need to. And now came the hard part.

"Michael, yes, it's Christine. Look I've got an opportunity to tape *Oprah* next Tuesday. They're working it out so it won't interfere with our makeovers . . ."

"Won't interfere? I don't see how it wouldn't interfere," Michael questioned me and I could tell by his bored "why are you bothering me with this?" tone of voice that he was not a happy executive producer.

"Really, I will be able to take our Tuesday makeover on the air in the morning, and then consult and organize everything for our Wednesday makeover before I leave. Amy's lined up, and I'll be on the phone with her throughout the day."

"I don't know. This takes away from our show and you know it's May sweeps and we do these makeovers for the ratings," Michael said.

"I promise you it won't interfere. I've done so many makeovers, and Amy has been there for most of them. I would never compromise the integrity of my work. You know that."

Because he knew my integrity and maybe a little because *Oprah* was an ABC show like *Live,* he reluctantly agreed. Even Michael knew everyone bowed to Oprah.

"Just don't let me know you're gone. I need everything covered," he said in his most irritated voice.

"Of course, Michael. You've got enough on your plate not to have to worry about the makeovers," I told him, making it all about him, just the way he liked it. Why should I think this time he would make it easy for me? Life for Michael is about making his world easy, at any and all costs.

And then it hit me. How would I make it all work?

The plane to Chicago took off right on time. The flight was smooth. My seatmate was an extremely tall man who had to fold his body into the business-class seat. I was determined not to make eye contact with him because I needed this time to relax. All I wanted was something to eat to calm my overmedicated nauseous stomach. He was determined to find out who I was and why I was going to Chicago. Oprah, as always, was the magic word, and over the minimal food service of peanuts and Diet Coke plus my much-needed pain pill he talked the entire trip, making me even more anxious because I needed to change my fashion focus from makeovers to appropriate dressing.

I got off the plane and quickly saw the driver holding a sign with my name on it. So far, so good, it was only a short thirty-minute ride to Harpo's studios. I closed my eyes and leaned my head back, trying to relax before I had to gear up again. My television makeup from this morning was now feeling caked and heavy. I wished I had taken it off before I left New York.

The driver startled me, "Sorry for the delay, seems to be an accident up ahead."

I glanced at the dashboard clock: two o'clock. I was supposed to be at the studio NOW.

"Yes, we're en route. Delay due to a traffic accident. ETA about thirty minutes," the driver talked into his pager.

THIRTY MINUTES. But I'm supposed to be there now.

"That was the studio wondering where we are," he informed me as if the timing was no big deal. "Don't worry, I'll have you there in no time," he assured me.

But I was not assured. He didn't have to change, redo makeup, or get briefed on the segment. He didn't have to appear on *Oprah*.

"We're still gathering some on-the-street tape of women wearing inappropriate clothing items. But don't worry, we'll have time to show you the tapes when you get here on Tuesday before we go on air," the producer told me the day before, when she was supposed to have copies of the tapes delivered to my New York hotel so I could look them over and have my thoughts ready before the show. Everyone says don't worry, so why was I so worried? Probably because I know live television. Once the cameras rolled I would be on my own, and now I wouldn't be prepared. Just the thought made me shake.

"We're right around the corner," the driver said into the pager. As we turned the corner I saw the door to Harpo Studios, a pacing intern impatiently waited.

"Ms. Kunzelman, please follow me. We need to hurry," she said, grabbing the garment bag out of my arms and marching ahead at a rapid speed. "The producer is waiting for you in the green room."

My stomach was in knots. My joints were protesting. I couldn't take any more pain medication and still be able to talk coherently on TV. My anxiety was at a dangerous level. My heart was beating as if it was going to come out of my chest. As we passed the studio I heard the audience clapping. The show was already in progress.

"Hi Christine, I'm Meg. We need to rush. The show has started. We're running a little ahead of schedule because Oprah has an event tonight."

"If I can just look at the tapes," I said in a nervous, high-pitched voice.

"No time, we need to get you touched up and on the set. Just watch the monitors and comment on what you see," she said, taking my arm and rushing me to the makeup room.

"I need to change first."

"No time, your outfit is fine," she said looking over my wrinkled dress from the *Live* show. "Beck, this is Christine. You have two minutes to touch her up."

Beck was calm and collected. I guess he was comfortable with two minutes to do hair and makeup. My lips quivered as he tried to apply fresh lip liner.

"Honey, hold still. You look great. Take a deep breath and keep those kissers in place for me." Two minutes later he was removing the plastic cape, brushing off my shoulders with one hand, and following me down the hall with his brush, comb, and hair spray, working on my hair as we made our way to the stage. In the wings, Beck continued his primping while Meg filled me in. I was trying hard to concentrate on what she said over the noise of the show now in progress.

"Christine, focus. Look at me. We're going to place you on the set during the next commercial. You'll be introduced, and we'll go right to the tape. Watch the monitor and comment on what you see, what you would change, why it's wrong. Just keep talking as the tape rolls," and she started walking me out onto the set.

"But we didn't discuss the tape, I have no idea what's on it, we didn't rehearse, we didn't talk through the segment, I'm coming into the middle of the show, I don't know who the other guests are or what they have already talked about . . ." I rattled on and on, my legs throbbing so intensely I didn't know if I could make it to the set.

"I'm sorry, this was out of my control," Meg shouted at me in a frustrated whisper. "We started early, you were late, just wing it for God's sake, just wing it."

Wing it? This is not a local TV show. This is *Oprah.* You don't wing it on *Oprah.*

Meg grabbed both of my shoulders, looked me squarely in the eyes, and said, "JUST WING IT." I knew the conversation was over. I knew I had to get focused and control my stomach. I was so queasy from all the medication and yet I hoped it was working so I could get through this. It was time.

The bright glare of the studio lights, the murmurs of the audience, the cameras, the stage manager with his headset and clipboard, and there they were, three yellow club chairs, two occupied by women I didn't know and a third one, empty, waiting for me. As I sat down, Beck sprayed my hair as if there was going to be a hurricane on the set. I was on the set of *Oprah,* with *Oprah* walking over to me as the stage manager counted down, "Four, three, two and . . ."

"Welcome back, we have Christine Kunzelman joining us. Christine is the author of *Quickstyle,* a terrific new book from Random House on accessorizing. Christine, what are the most obvious mistakes women make in dressing appropriate?" Oprah asked in her best girlfriend-to-girlfriend manner.

But where was the monitor, where was the tape? Panic set in as I saw the red light on the camera pointed right at me. My fashion experience kicked in full gear and I started talking about inappropriate dressing. Smiling, radiating into the camera just like my television coach taught me many years ago. Out of the corner of my eye I saw my producer Meg, frantically, hysterically waving her hands toward a nearby TV monitor. Two young interns held up quickly scribbled cue cards:

Tape on monitor
Go To Monitor !!
MONITOR!!!!!!!!!!

And there it was, over in the corner, a TV monitor with clips of women on the street in inappropriate clothing. Rolling along at its own pace while I was talking about something totally different. Trying to recover quickly I changed gears, "Light-color pants should always be on the looser side," I said, trying to lower my nervous high-pitched voice. Then the two other guests, who had so far sat in total silence, amazed at what was going on all around them, decided to chime in and we all started talking at once as the tape rolled on and on. Oprah quickly called for a commercial before we self-imploded on her exquisite yellow chairs.

Meg ran over to me, "Didn't you see the monitor?"

"How could I see it, it's over in the corner with people all around it," I said, thinking at any moment I would lose my digested pain pills, airplane peanuts, and Diet Coke on the set of *Oprah*.

"Five, four, three, two and . . ." The stage manager counted down, clearing the set.

"Welcome back," Oprah said. "Let's change gears a bit."

I thought, "Oh yes, let's change everything." There I sat with two women who were also experts but I had no idea in what. A pacing producer whispered into her headset, probably to defend herself to her executive producer who was in the booth going crazy that a tape was rolling on the screen as I talked about something else. Like listening to sound from one show while watching pictures from another, only unfortunately it was on the same show.

But Oprah, being Oprah, started talking about women squeezing into too small a size and all her experts, myself included, jumped in with strong opinions of right and wrong. Luckily for me, Oprah liked my opinion that it wasn't about size, it was about fit.

"She used to be a size four and she's going to be a size 4 regardless of how it fits her, armpits hanging out and all," Oprah demonstrated with her arms in a swinging position.

"Exactly, Oprah, we care more about the size than the fit. If we wore a size ten five years ago we want to wear a size ten today, regardless of how we're squeezed in," I said, my voice now strong and controlled.

Oprah and I talked, on national television, my overly sprayed helmet hair not moving as I nodded and agreed, adding information here and there while the two other experts sat silently. It was just Oprah and me. Chatting like girlfriends over coffee. Oprah had saved my day.

Meg stopped pacing and talking into her headset.

The interns were no longer holding cue cards.

The audience sat mesmerized.

And my stomach relaxed, my peanuts and Diet Coke intact. The Oprah adrenaline was in full force, and for a few moments I forgot about RA. Talking to Oprah really was like talking to my best friend, and, in this case, it was like talking to a friend who knew I was in trouble and was there to bail me out.

When a TV show taping is over, it is over. The audience is quickly moved out. The bright lights dimmed. The host magically disappears, and the guests are promptly led back to their dressing rooms to pack up and move out. Cars wait outside to take them to their next destination. But this time, they couldn't end it fast enough, because they were already working on the next show. This show was in the can, and everyone involved was done with it. When you were new in television it could be shattering. A quick "good job" if you're lucky but most of the time just a hasty "thanks." It was very anticlimactic after the adrenaline rush of the show. I asked if I could thank Oprah, and my producer Meg looked at me as if I was asking her to personally drive me back to New York. "Oprah is already out of the building," she informed me, as she waited impatiently for me to gather my things. "Becca, please get Christine to her car," Meg grabbed a young intern who walked by. "I have to get back to work," she said leaving the room.

"I should say good-bye to the other experts," I said to the pacing intern. "I really never got to talk to them." "Oh, they left," she answered. Of course, everyone had left.

Back in the car riding to O'Hare I realized I had not spoken to Amy all day. It was now six o'clock. Not sure if this was a good sign or a bad one, I dialed her number.

"How's it going?" I shouted into the phone, hearing the background noise of blow dryers in the New York salon.

"Going good, how was *Oprah*?" she shouted back.

"A long story that I will share with you later. Did they get the auburn color for her hair?"

"Yes, it looks good. I checked it under the spotlights in the salon to make sure it's not too red. They're blow-drying her right now," Amy said in a relaxed tone that confirmed everything was fine. "You have a safe flight and relax. This has been a crazy day for you. I'll see you in the morning."

"Thanks Amy, you've been great. See you tomorrow."

I had pushed my RA to the back of my mind during *Oprah* in order to get the job done. Between the adrenaline rush of live television and my controlling need for professionalism, I was able to do this. But now, back at the hotel, relief and fatigue took over.

I wanted to call Shelly and tell him about the show. I tried to reach for the phone on the nightstand, but my hands and arms were too weak to even support the handset, making me get up and lift the phone onto the bed. It was all I could do to hold the receiver to my ear.

"Hi, gorgeous, I've been waiting to hear from you. How was your flight to Chicago?" Shelly asked.

"You would have loved to be in my seat. Some athlete was sitting next to me. He had a big Superbowl ring and was so tall he could hardly get his legs behind the seat in front. The flight attendant called him Mr. Frazer."

"Frazer? It had to be Walt Frazer from the New York Knicks. That was an NBA championship ring! He's an All-Star. I would have loved to have been on your flight."

"And Oprah, wait till you hear about the show . . ." I interjected, reaching for a pain pill to dull the stress that the day had taken on my joints. The adrenaline was gone, the reality back in full force.

"Walt Frazer was one of my favorite players when I lived in New York. Did you tell him I'm a Knicks fan?"

We continued talking about Walt and the Knicks. Shelly dealt with major problems all day long. His escape was talking sports, and after the day I had it was fine with me.

"Oh, how was your *Oprah* segment?" he finally asked.

"Great, just great."

14

Rejected for the Rat Cage

After a frustrating summer experimenting with various combinations of the same drugs, my RA was no better. We were in Laguna, where we had a getaway town house. What better place to spend Thanksgiving we thought, making our holiday plans. We didn't factor in spending part of it in the emergency room at the Laguna Beach Hospital after a call from Dr. Kalunian.

"Sorry to call on a holiday, but I got your labs back and your liver functions are elevated again, this time even higher. You need to get to a lab and take them again."

"But it's a holiday," I said, trying to figure out how I would juggle my houseguests and my lab work.

"Go to the emergency room, and have them fax the results over to me. This is important. You need to get right on it," Dr. Kalunian insisted. Dr. Kalunian was not an alarmist, but he was very conservative when it came to health. It seemed as if I was always redoing lab work.

Shelly and I drove to the emergency room, leaving family and out-of-town guests at home thinking we had a business emergency. Thank God everyone was busy catching up and didn't ask what kind of emergency. At the hospital, the ER was packed with crying babies and sick-looking people. One young boy sat waiting to be seen with blood dripping through a make-shift bandage on his arm.

Five hours later we left, with corrected and more positive lab results in hand. Now if only the turkey in the oven was doing as well.

A week later I was on my way to UCLA. I had a ten o'clock appointment at the research center. I had waited for this appointment for months. It felt like the only hope I had left. Today I would find out what it was like to be a medical lab rat.

"Christine, we have to keep you going until this new group of TNF drugs becomes available. They look promising," Dr. Kalunian told me over and over when I lost hope, which over the past few years was often. He even set up the appointment at the London hospital, when in desperation Shelly and I visited in hopes of getting into their research program. In a thick British accent the doctor informed me in no uncertain terms that I was ineligible for a London trial when I was a U.S. citizen. He thought I was coming for another opinion. Dr. Wallace had said beg, borrow, or steal to get the new drugs, but in this foreign environment, with a doctor who looked at me like "why did you make this trip?" I knew that all options were off the table. I would have to wait until testing happened in the United States.

Finally, back at UCLA, the testing was under way and I was desperate to be a part of it. UCLA had the new TNF-blocking drug, Enbrel, that I had unsuccessfully tried to get first from the manufacturer and then from the research program in London. TNF stands for Tumor Necrosis Factor, a normal protein that plays a role in the immune system. Patients with rheumatoid arthritis usually have too much TNF, which causes inflammation, and that can compromise the immune systems. Enbrel was one of the first drugs being tested that offered the hope of reducing TNF levels.

Dr. Kalunian had set up the meeting. The research center was a few streets off the main campus of UCLA. Driving up to the address I saw an old building squeezed in between a fire station and the veterans' cemetery. Once inside I realized the outside looked new compared to the sterile, crumbling interior. The waiting room had furniture that had to be from the sixties and tattered medical brochures that had been read too many times. I didn't care. Enbrel might be the new miracle drug. I was in dire need of a miracle.

"Christine Schwab?" the assistant called as she walked into the reception room where I was the only patient.

"Good morning," I answered with all the positive energy I felt.

"Fill out these papers and Dr. Bulpitt will be with you shortly," said the nurse as she handed me a thick stack of questions about my health.

How long does it take me to get dressed in the morning? On a good day, no time at all. On a bad day, way too long.

Did I need help? My pride would never let me ask for help. I was not old.

Could I open jars by myself? No, Shelly knew to open my jars so I never had to ask.

Where on a scale of one to one hundred would I rate my daily pain? It was all over the place. I guess I would rate my average day of pain around eighty five.

On that same scale where was I emotionally? Much lower than I would ever let on.

Did I believe I could be helped with medications? Yes, with THIS new medicine. I had given up hope on all the others.

I took my list of medications out of my purse and began, prepared for what would be one of the most important days of my life. Azulfidine, methotrexate, oral gold, imuran, Plaquenil, Cytoxan, cyclosporine, penicillamine, steroids, and Azulfidine again. Seven years of toxic drugs that either didn't work or worked but with complications too severe for me to continue taking them.

The assistant escorted me to an examining room, even more dismal than the waiting room. The only place for me to sit was on a cold, steel exam table. Everything in the room was white, beige, or green, but over the years it had all turned gray, even the pillowcase on the worn, flat pillow for my head.

In walked Dr. Bulpitt, a tall, imposing man in his mid-thirties. Between the two of us, we took up almost every inch of space in the room. He carried my thick, six-year UCLA medical chart, and the questionnaires I had just filled out. We sat facing each other, me on the bed with my legs hanging over the side, he on the small rolling stool in front of me. I went into my full-blown sales mode about how glad I was to be here. How I went to London to try to get TNF only to be rejected because I was a U.S. citizen. I chatted nonstop about my up-and-down journey with RA. This man had medicine that I needed. This man would determine if I was accepted in the program.

He sat there listening, no readable expression on his face. The more he listened, the more I talked, in rapid, anxious sentences. I knew how to sell, and today I was selling my body for research, willingly.

Who knew the risks? I was beyond caring. I had lost the quality of my life. The fear of my disease being revealed had shaken my professional confidence. Something on Dr. Bulpitt's face told me he wasn't hearing me. His acknowledging nods of the head were polite but not absorbed. I stopped the sales pitch.

"Christine, I'm sorry you had to come here today. Had I read your chart earlier I would have called you and canceled. You're not a candidate for this research program. You've been treated unsuccessfully on too many drugs. We need patients who have only been on a few drugs, because we need positive results."

My brain heard what he said but my heart couldn't believe it.

"But I'm a compliant patient. I have a great attitude. I know I'll do well in the program. I've been waiting for years . . ."

In a quiet, nonemotional voice Dr. Bulpitt continued. "I'm sure you are, but we only have so many openings, and you're too risky. You have failed on too many drugs. If you fail on this drug it lowers the chance of the FDA approving it. FDA approval would allow it to help millions. The animal research so far has been very positive. We can't risk you lowering the odds."

"But that's exactly why I need this." By now I was pleading. "I have to get in this program. Dr. Kalunian has told me about TNF for years. I've waited for years. I tried to get it from the manufacturer. I even went to London to try to get into a human research program. Please . . ."

Dr. Bulpitt never changed his expressionless face. To him I was one of the experimental rats in the cages, one that didn't make the cut.

"I'm sorry. Like I said, I wish I'd looked at your chart earlier. I could have saved you the trip."

I felt the tears well up. I saw on his face that it didn't matter what I said or how I begged. He was a research doctor; it was all about numbers and stats. He didn't see me as a person, a desperate person. He saw me as a patient who most likely wouldn't do well in his new test. I was tainted with dozens of combinations of drugs that UCLA doctors had given me over the past seven years. Drugs that had played havoc with my life and failed, and now that failure would prevent me from a drug that could potentially help. Where was the fairness in this? My built-up hopes and frustrations burst out in tears as I grabbed my purse and ran out the door, down the hallways, and out to the parking lot. I sat in my car for twenty minutes, trying to stop crying and to figure out how it all went so wrong. I felt hopeless.

Dr. Kalunian's answer machine picked up after the first ring, indicating that he was on another line. I waited for the beep, "Dr. Kalunian, Christine Schwab, I just left Dr. Bulpitt's office, and he said I'm not a candidate for the research program because

I have failed with too many drugs," my voice cracked as I choked out the painful words.

My phone rang before I could even start my car: "Christine, Ken Kalunian. I'm so sorry. Just hold on, let me see what I can do. I'll get back to you."

I couldn't gather any hope or enthusiasm. How could I tell Shelly? His expectations were as high as mine. Together we waited for this day, this opportunity. What did I do now? I left all my hope in that dismal research building. A wave of depression froze me behind the wheel of my car. I couldn't even turn the key in my ignition. I didn't know where to go and so I sat in the parking lot as people drove in and out. People filled with hopes and fears, looking for answers. Patients involved in the many research programs going on in the building, offering hope that I had been denied.

I cried myself into a stupor, then into sleep. Just like my childhood, enough tears, and I could put myself to sleep where the pain wasn't as intense, if only for a short time. My phone woke me up.

"Sweetie, I thought you were going to call me after your appointment. How did it go?" Shelly asked. Looking at the clock on my dashboard I realized I had been sleeping in my car for almost an hour.

"I'm not a candidate for the program. I've been on too many drugs and failed. They want people who will get good results," I answered, all the emotion drained from my voice and dried up like the streaked tears on my face.

"Oh, Christine," was all Shelly could say. He held as much hope as I did. He went to London with me to try to get TNF. He helped me write my pleading letter to the manufacturer trying to get into the early research. "Where are you?"

"I'm in the parking lot."

"At UCLA?" he asked.

"Yes, at the Veteran building."

"Let's meet at the Hamlet Gardens and have lunch and talk this through. I can be there in thirty minutes," he said with forced optimism.

"No, I'm not hungry, I think I'll go home. You don't have to come all the way over the hill from the valley, we'll talk tonight," I said, trying to sound positive.

"You have to eat. I'll see you at Hamlet Gardens. Get a table and order some wine. Christine, I love you, we'll be okay."

I wasn't so sure. Chronic pain wears on a person. I could see it in my face even if others couldn't. My skills with makeup helped cover the signs of pain. A sparkling eye shadow will draw attention away—I had taught that to all my viewers—now I used it for myself. Almost seven years of chronic pain. Almost seven years of hopes and dreams dashed with failed drugs. Complications of thinning hair, hearing loss, and a constant sensitive stomach were reminders. The biggest reminder of all was the daily pain of moving from place to place. My feet, knees, shoulders, elbows, wrists, and hand joints were now inflamed, ravaged by RA. The hope of the research program had kept me going. Hope kept my fantasy world alive enough to move me forward. And now that hope was gone. Hamlet Gardens, right around the corner from UCLA, was one of our favorites. Fresh guacamole made right at your table. We had celebrated many events there, enjoyed many pre–Geffen Playhouse dinners. I could leave my car in this lot and walk, it was that close. Shelly had to drive all the way from his office at Universal Studios in Studio City. In a trance I got out of my car, locked the door, and slowly walked toward the restaurant.

How would we be okay? Shelly never lost hope as each year of living with RA took its toll on my body and my mind. He was the one who kept me going, moving forward, searching for answers. How could we be okay when I had lost all hope? When the only answers now were different combinations of drugs that have already failed me or desperate, questionable, unorthodox treatments like draining and cleaning my blood or healers who ran their hands over my body making vibrations that had no logical origin. My reflection in the passing store windows was of a tired, worn-down, defeated woman. What happened to the vibrant, healthy, energetic television reporter? What happened to the healthy, toned, and exciting woman my husband married?

15

Just Do It . . .

I swallowed the pain pill with a glass of water as I sat in the plush chairs of the American Airlines Admirals Club, watching the beehive of activity as businesspeople worked on computers and cell phones arranging their work schedules while we all waited to board our planes. Shelly and I were headed to New York for a hectic week of work. I wondered how I would get through it. My new regime of medications was yet another combination of old drugs, the hope being that the new combination would make the old ineffective drugs work. Sort of like rearranging old furniture in the same room in the hopes that it will look new. Dr. Kalunian tried to keep me encouraged that it was just a matter of finding the right combination for me. I was still feeling the rejection of being too tainted by failed drugs to be a candidate for the research program. I tried to figure out how I could maneuver through the New York week, both with my attitude and my pain, and for once I couldn't come up with any new answers to my old problems.

As Shelly read the paper I sipped lukewarm coffee and ate a miniature bagel to coat my stomach for the pain pill.

"Do you have RA?" a husky voice startled me out of my daze. Before me stood a tall, attractive, imposing woman, scrolling her eyes down to my trendy, animal-print sneakers.

All I could respond, as I slowly got my joints moving to stand up, now face-to-face with her, was, *"What?"*

"Do you have rheumatoid arthritis?" she repeated in a louder, deeper voice.

Startled, I looked around to see if anyone had heard. The room was filled with industry people, people who couldn't know my secret.

"I've been watching you, how slowly you move to get up and then I saw your sneakers and I had to ask because you look like you have RA," she rattled on, inspecting me for damage as if I were a rental car with potential dents being returned to Hertz. All that was missing was a checklist: steroid moon-shaped face—check, damage to hands—not visible, feet—hidden. Now face-to-face I recognized it was the actress Kathleen Turner. Why was she in my face about RA? I glanced around the room again, expecting to see secret agents talking to each other on their hidden microphones, "Yep, got another one, RA for sure."

"The reason I'm asking," she continued in that sexy voice that is so recognizable, now standing so close to me that I feared our noses would touch if she moved in any more, "is because I have RA. What medications are you taking? You look pretty stiff."

Kathleen Turner has RA? The sexy star of the movie *Body Heat*. This gorgeous woman right in front of me. "I'm over doctors, I finally got some relief by going to Mexico. Now I grind up animal bones and drink their tea and I'm better. Have you tried that?" she continued in rapid speed. "I think it's working."

Ground-up animal bones? Mexico? Confronted in public? If Kathleen Turner recognized my RA, do others as well? My head was whirling.

"I'm in the process of trying new combinations of old drugs. My doctor said we just have to keep me going until the new drugs that are being tested are available. They're testing at UCLA right now, so it's only a matter of time."

"Ugh, doctors, conventional medicines, I've had it. Really you should try something else, it doesn't look like what you're doing is helping. Cool sneakers, your feet a problem?"

Shelly, newspapers and carry-on in hand, interrupted our conversation. "Christine, we have to board," he said as he took my arm. He could tell that whatever she was saying to me was traumatic. "That was Kathleen Turner," I said as we moved toward the boarding gate. "She has RA."

"She told you?" Shelly asked.

"She recognized that I have RA from my sneakers and the way I walked."

He didn't say any more. He saw the fear on my face.

I leaned my head back in my plane seat and fell into a fitful sleep. Chicken bones, dog bones, cat bones. Kathleen Turner on the kitchen table having wild sex with William Hurt in the movie *Body Heat,* steam coming from a brewing pot on the stove. As I started to sip the smelly brew I woke up. If Kathleen Turner could recognize my disease, how many others knew? Was my secret about to become public?

But I quickly forgot about those concerns when I got a call from the UCLA research lab as we were being driven into New York City. Could I come in next week to start the trial testing on Enbrel? I didn't know what happened. I didn't want to tell them that I had been rejected, so I called Dr. Kalunian.

"Congratulations, Christine, that's great news," he said in his busy, behind-schedule voice.

"Do you know what happened, why I'm now accepted?" I asked, almost afraid of the answer, hoping it wasn't a mistake.

"Just go and enroll. This is your chance, don't ask any questions, just do it. Gotta run, good news, Christine," and he was gone. As I hung up the phone part of my mind asked what happened. The other part repeated his words, "Just do it." And I did.

The research room in the rheumatology building at UCLA is the last stop for patients who have tried everything else to no avail. It's a somber place. There's not a lot of smiling. These patients are tired, worn down, and sick.

I walked in and sat down on the only empty Barcalounger-type chair. One young woman looked like she was asleep as an IV pumped trial medications into her arm. Even in her sleep, her mouth was down-turned, defeated. Another older woman was complaining to the technician nonstop, nothing was right, she hurt everywhere, nothing was working. She glanced at me with a look that said, "Just wait."

I filled out paper after paper until my swollen, inflamed fingers cramped from holding the pen. I signed away my life. I would hold them responsible for nothing, I was now on my own, floating, without a life vest, in the UCLA research lake, grasping at a floating tree branch that was just beyond my reach as I realized I was treading water way over my head.

"You have to stop all your medications for RA as of today. We need to cleanse your system before we start the test," the technician told me in a distant "don't get attached" voice. All of my medications? I would be taking nothing to relieve my pain? The thought petrified me. For the past seven years I had been living on medications, but I signed the form. "Just do it," Dr. Kalunian's words, echoed in my head.

"We'll call you when your trial kit comes in. Remember, no drugs," the technician said, moving on to take the IV out of the sleeping patient's arm.

I looked back at the room as I walked out. There was nothing warm or comforting in there. It was a sterile, serious environment. Even the air seemed still. The only thing missing were the rat cages. They were in the next room, already moving on to test a new drug. For a minute fear overtook my feeling of hope. What was ahead?

16
And the Results Are . . .

I glanced over at my day planner sitting next to me on the couch in my den, waiting for me to fill in all the blank squares. The calendar was open to September. I'd drawn a large red circle around September 25th, with "UCLA" inside. Nine months. I had been in the UCLA Enbrel research testing program for nine months. I had completed my last set of labs for the double-blind study a few weeks ago. Now on my couch, watching daytime television, wrapped in my afghan, I was waiting for the phone call that would tell me if I had been on the placebo, half strength, or full strength. My guess was that I was on half strength. The biggest news would be when would I get my new Enbrel kit with the full dosage of medicine. I had stayed the course when others had dropped out. I would soon be rewarded.

While reruns of *Friends* played on TV, the scenario of the last nine months played over and over in my head. I flipped the pages of my day planner, my UCLA appointments entered in red pen and my work schedule in blue. With each month, there were more red boxes and fewer blue boxes. The travel boxes, in green, had almost stopped. I had become a prisoner of my disease. I was held hostage in a research program.

I entered the program in January 1997. It was a double-blind study, meaning no one except the drug company representatives knew whether patients were on a placebo, half-strength, or full-strength doses of the new medication.

I always had the same UCLA lab technician, Tina, a petite, struggling young mom with long, curly hair like Amy Irving's. She was professional, never giving hope but never giving up on hope. She answered what questions she could, avoiding any that might give away too much information. Because of the double-blind study, neither she, nor my doctor, knew what dosage—if any—I was on so she couldn't have shared anything if she wanted to.

I had waited so long for this new line of drugs to become available, so I had to be positive—"Sparkle Plenty"—that I would be one of the lucky ones getting a full dosage of Enbrel in my twice-weekly shots. Even in that sad lab room at UCLA, I kept my hope alive.

I was rewarded with six months of feeling good. Not just good, great. As if the disease had been lifted out of my body. I had energy, not steroid-induced energy, but my old, healthy energy. My joints felt almost normal, I could move around without grimacing. I could get out of bed in the morning without feeling like a stiff cardboard cutout of myself. Enbrel was the magic drug, my ticket out of chronic illness and back to my former life. I was ecstatic.

Then Tina brought me back to reality. "Your sed rate (the rate that indicates inflammation in the body) is starting to rise." My labs had been good for six months, so this negative news was jarring. I equated sed rate with pain. Before the research program, the higher the sed rate, the more intense the pain.

"Is this happening to any of the other study participants? How are they doing?" I was always asking about the others, how was their health, who had left the program, who was still in. Tina, protecting privacy, identified the patients by location.

"The woman from Dallas left the program, sure that she was on the placebo. Between the travel back and forth to UCLA and the lack of results she finally gave up. The man from Orange County quit last week, sure that he felt he was on a half dosage. He couldn't take the pain anymore. About a third of the participants have left, some frightened by the revelations of a few patients dying or being diagnosed with some type of cancer. They read the updates and consent forms as the study progressed and even though we told them these issues most likely were not caused by the drug, their fear takes over. They won't sign the forms, so they have to leave the program," Tina said.

"I must be on the half strength. I thought it was the full strength before, but now with my sed rate going up and pain returning to my joints I'm sure I have the half dosage," I said, looking at Tina for clarification. She didn't answer. She couldn't. So why did I keep prodding? Because the fear of having the disease return petrified me, taking me back to that dark, powerless place where my life spun out of control.

And then my health went into a tailspin. Almost overnight I watched my hands age. Knobby knuckles popped out like tiny balls hidden under the skin of each joint, stretching the skin like a double bedsheet pulled over a queen-size mattress. Then my fingers started slanting outward, as if reaching for something to the side of my pinkies. I looked like the cover photo of the arthritis pamphlets in the doctor's office. My worst nightmare.

My feet blew up red and swollen and I couldn't squeeze into anything but sneakers, flip-flops, or slippers. I was in my early forties and dressing more like a mall walker on leave from her assisted-living home than a fashion reporter. Once again my wardrobe of heeled shoes was gathering dust.

"Please, just a few steroids to get me through this *Entertainment Tonight* piece, just for the day before and of the shoot, that's all I need, so I can walk, talk, and stand like a seminormal person," I pleaded with Dr. Kalunian, showing up at his office one morning, unannounced, in desperate need of help. I was beginning to sound like an addict.

"Christine, you're now under Dr. Bulpitt's care in the research program. I can't give you anything. I'm sorry, I understand your predicament, but these are the rules of pharmaceutical trials, I can't break them," he said with his hand on the knob of the exam room door, eager to get away from my neediness and on to his scheduled patients.

The next morning, after some frustrated tears in the shower, I took Tylenol and did the segment. I had to. What would I be, who would I be if I wasn't on TV? My identity was tied up in my fantasy job. The fantasy that consumed my life as a child continued on in adulthood, filling in the gaps of my insecurities. In television I was validated. I was no longer that little girl who always seemed to be seeking a place where she wasn't in the way. A place where she was appreciated. I had finally found my place. I finally saw myself as a whole person on the inside and the outside. Shelly had always recognized that in me, but it took me much longer to get to the same place. Now that person was crumbling. I thought I could deal by using my cocoon of denial, but the visible evidence now eradicated that. Once again, I was powerless. I no longer knew who I was.

Watching the *ET* segment air the next night, I wondered if I was the only person who could see the strain and pain on my face. I tried to give myself a pep talk, "You look fine, nobody is noticing the strain around your eyes." "Don't be so critical, everyone's watching the story, not you." "You know how you're feeling, everyone else is looking at your awesome Jil Sander jacket." But my pep talks to myself didn't work.

"You look fine, just more like a serious journalist," my husband said, addressing my concerns. "Like you could be on *60 Minutes* instead of *Entertainment Tonight*. You're too self-conscious. Only you would recognize the pain on your face."

Shelly always made me feel better, even though I knew he was lying. I looked tired and worn out. I looked old.

Finally it was September, the month of truth when the research envelopes would be opened and the results revealed. I still thought I was on the half dosage because of the relief I'd felt during the first six months of the study. That meant that once I got the full dosage, a reward for staying in the program, I would have my pre-RA life back. I couldn't wait.

It was difficult those last two months of the program, knowing that my RA was active and whatever dosage of medicine I was on was not working. I eliminated what travel and jobs I could and, with the aid of many assistants, plus a lot of downtime on the couch, which took my income from the green column to the red, I had survived.

The call came from Dr. Bulpitt in the afternoon of September 27nd. I was still in my pajamas and robe, my new uniform of choice

"Dr. Bulpitt here. The double-blind study is over and you were on the placebo," he said, as if he were telling me that the weather today would be seventy-two and sunny.

"Placebo?" Did that really mean I had not had any medicine in my body for the last nine months? I couldn't even grasp the doctor's words. And then I looked down in my lap at my swollen, slanted hands, grasping each other as if holding on for dear life. The pain had come back the last few months. The aches, the swelling, the fatigue, but I never let my mind go to the place of "placebo." And now I was hearing the word for the first time and I just couldn't get it to register. I looked into the mouthpiece of the phone as if the real truth was buried there and at any minute he would say something funny like "gotcha," but who was I kidding? I think Dr. Bulpitt has lost his sense of humor in one of his research projects. "What about how great I felt the first five months?" I asked, still trying to make sense of his words.

"Most likely, after seven years of so many toxic drugs, your body was responding to the elimination of drugs, making you feel healthy until all the drugs were out of your system. Then the inflammation returned." Not a positive note in his voice, not a concerned word, just the facts, the cold, shocking facts.

"So because I didn't have any drugs in my body I felt normal for awhile?" I asked again, still not comprehending how this could be possible.

"It's not unusual for a person who has taken large quantities of medications to feel somewhat better when all medications are withheld," Dr. Bulpitt said. He always sounded like he was reading a textbook to a group of med students, instead of trying to console a stressed patient.

"The good news is because you stayed in the program, you're eligible for the new Enbrel kit that will contain the full dosage of the medication. The final part of the testing will be with the remaining participants all on full-strength medication. We'll monitor you closely to make sure you can tolerate the drug."

Did he sound reserved? Was he giving me a heads-up that the drug might make me sick, maybe put me in the hospital like Methotrexate? Or was it my imagination? Part of me felt ecstatic that I could now have the real deal going into my body instead of purified water. The other part of me felt the same fear I felt when signing the papers for the initial testing. How would my body react? Would this be the miracle drug that would put me in remission or another toxic drug that would take me back to Cedars? All this time I was so sure I had the half dosage and that the full dosage would be incredible, only to find out that I was back at square one again. Nine months wasted. Nine months of devastation to my hands, now visibly disfigured. At least when I was on the steroids they kept the inflammation down. Inflammation, when out of control, means damage to the joints, some visible, some not. My fear of visible evidence of my disease was now a reality.

"Can I come in today?" I asked, my mind filled with conflicting thoughts.

"We'll have to call you when the kits come in, probably a week or two," Dr. Bulpitt said, eager to get off the phone. His five minutes of patience with me was nearing the end.

"But the people who were on the full dosage, they're doing great, right?" I said.

"Most of them are doing well. The drug looks positive."

And that was all I had to hear. Positive. I knew I would be one of the positive ones. I had waited almost eight years for relief. I would wait a little longer.

The only thing I wanted to do was climb in bed and try to process this information. I put a bottle of celebratory champagne in the refrigerator to chill, knowing that when Shelly got home, he would be eager for my news. I wouldn't let on about my fears of starting over. I didn't want to tell him about the placebo on the phone and, in the hectic rush of his day, he hadn't called. Buried safely under the comforter of my bed I had the afternoon to think. I came to the conclusion that even though I had damage to my hands as a result of being on the placebo, I had stayed the course, and now I would get the full strength of the drug. I gathered all my Sparkle Plenty abilities to turn this into a positive. I convinced myself that once on the real Enbrel, I would go into remission. Positive thoughts filled my head as I slipped off into a peaceful nap.

After a quick shower to wake up, I dressed in my best black cocktail dress, the Donna Karan with the very sheer skirt and the long jacket that made me feel sexy because of the illusion of being somewhat naked. On my feet, I wore my real ballet flats— ballet flats were out of style, but since they were the only shoes I could wear to a cocktail party, I went to the dance store and bought the real deal. My black lace fingerless gloves sat waiting on top of my beaded evening bag, ready to take us to the Universal charity dinner honoring Steven Spielberg at the

Century Plaza Hotel. Fingerless gloves were another new addition to my wardrobe, combining style with function. They covered the knobby part of my knuckles and helped hide the outward slant of my fingers. After seeing several pictures of myself holding a cocktail glass, hands slanted and distorted, I stopped drinking in public until I came across the glove solution.

Shelly walked in the door, pulling his tie off as he entered. He immediately saw the champagne bucket. "We're celebrating?" he asked.

"Yes, the news from the research program," I said, handing him the champagne to open and giving him a kiss.

"It must be good, you're smiling," he said, popping the cork and filling our glasses. The music of Vivaldi's *Four Seasons* played in the background as I explained the test results. Shelly looked confused about how I could be so happy when I not only hadn't been on any medicine, but now would have to start over to find out if the medicine would even work for me.

"I know it sounds crazy, but just the fact that I stayed in the program means I will get this medicine years before the public. It's a chance, it's hope, Shelly, and I am so in need of hope." He got that. We toasted the nine-month birth of hope. Shelly changed his clothes for the evening while I sat sipping my champagne, looking at my reflection in the mirrored walls of our living room. I looked young again, not the tired and drained woman of the past months. It wasn't an extra layer of cover-up, an added line of blue pencil inside my eyes to make them sparkle or a salon facial looking back at me. It was the amazing antiaging effects of hope.

17

The Robo Arm Makeover

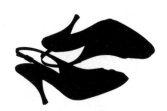

My antiaging process was short-lived. A month later in New York it was reality-check time.

"You look like you've been working hard," my producer at *Live* told me as we sat in the early morning hours on the stools that Regis and Kathie Lee would later occupy. It was code for: "You look like hell." I had noticed people looking at me with more intensity, but this was the first in-my-face confrontation and it shook me to my already fragile core. Was my replacement waiting in the shadows? I had to stop myself from glancing back toward the studio wings. We were rehearsing a fall fashion segment with models and props. The runway music blared as the director communicated with me through the studio loudspeaker, going over my talking points and the order of the models.

"It's been crazy in the dressing room this morning, and I only had time to do half my face, and, you know, the lights in this studio are notorious for making everyone look tired," I explained, trying to balance my first cup of coffee with my note cards in my lap, all the time keeping the palms of my hands turned up to hide their distortion.

"You're right," my producer kindly agreed, "everyone is constantly complaining, some celebrities won't come on the show unless they can bring their own lighting man to add a 'fill' light." A fill light is placed on the floor and shines up into their faces, filling in all the crevices that are created by either bad overhead lighting, or in some cases, simply age. But a glimpse at myself in the many television monitors placed all over the studio told me I needed more than a fill light. I was not looking good. What I didn't tell her was that morning I was unable to lift my arms up high enough to wash my hair, being forced once again to use dry shampoo. My puffy eyes were now framed by dull and lifeless hair. I made a mental note to ask the show's makeup artist to spend extra time hiding my puffy eyes.

It had been almost a month since Dr. Bulpitt's call. Between paperwork and the politics at UCLA it was one delay after another to start the Enbrel. Nobody had a straight answer. "Shouldn't be much longer" and "just be patient" were the only communications that came my way. Part of me wanted to lash out with anger. But as in my childhood, my rages remained silent. I was afraid that if I spoke up I might be labeled a nuisance and someone would withhold my Enbrel kit and with it, my chance at returning to a normal life. Survival. I had to maintain a survival mode. I had to keep my frustrations hidden.

With Mama Dorothy I'd learned to accept what I had and keep my anger inside. If I expressed discontent, I risked upsetting Mama Dorothy and then I might have to move to another home. Life at Mama Dorothy's wasn't good, but the fear of moving to another unknown home was worse. And so for me rage was a silent, internal emotion. Mama Dorothy wasn't even aware that I was angry or that I would have any cause to be. And, she didn't care anyway. Her priorities were enforcing strict rules to keep some type of order in the house, and making sure the monthly checks came in on time. My only concern was surviving until the next visit with my mom.

Now I had to rely on the skills I honed at Mama Dorothy's. I would be a good girl, waiting patiently—at least on the outside.

On the inside my fears raged. Damage continued to my unmedicated body. My hands were slanting more, my feet were aching, and I couldn't use my knees to sit or stand without feeling the most excruciating agony radiate from them into my entire body. Before RA, I never realized knee joints were indispensable in just moving around every day. I tried to figure out every way possible to not involve knee movement. Could I pee standing up in the shower? Revolting. So I drank fewer liquids because then I wouldn't have to lower myself to the toilet seat as often, now seemingly miles away from a standing position. As I inched myself toward the toilet seat my knee bones seemed to catch in their hinges. Each small bend felt like it forced the hinge open a little more. My fear was that my knees would explode, tearing away from their sockets, and I would end up in a wheelchair, just like my mom predicted. A raised seat was totally out of the question unless absolutely mandatory. Altered bathrooms were for the aged, not for me. Keeping my body stiff, I could lower myself onto the couch by just falling backward, no knees even needed. Chairs were eliminated whenever possible. Even I couldn't figure out how to fall into a chair without toppling over, and believe me, I tried. Of course, all of these solutions only worked when I was alone, safe from prying eyes. Nobody to stare at my damaged hands, or to see me fall into a couch. It was safer for me to be alone during the day. At night I begged out of some industry events when I could. Other times I had to suck it up and go, gloved, in my ballet flats, hiding my pain with a Sparkle Plenty face and a pain pill. Surely God was testing me. But why was it taking so long?

Control. Today I was desperate for some type of control. As a child I took control by escaping into a pretend world I found in the many books I read. I watched my mom take control by buying me a new dress or getting my hair cut. Even the simplest thing like polishing my fingernails in ballerina pink made my mom feel like she was in control of me. For the past seven years, living with RA and working in the television field where control was in the hands of the producers and executives, the only thing I could control was my appearance through makeup and style. Now, looking at my damaged hands, even that seemed to have escaped me.

Dr. Kalunian had mentioned a leading hand surgeon at Cedars who might be able to help me, and today I needed help, even if it came in the form of surgery. I called and took the first available appointment for a consultation. If there was a rewards program for frequent doctor visits, I would be collecting points to exchange for some exotic trip. Unfortunately, all I was collecting was expensive Beverly Hills and Westwood parking receipts.

After two young doctors in training pulled, squeezed, and diagrammed my hands, the surgeon came in. I knew he was important from the way the young doctors scurried to the corners of the room, charts in hand.

With a gentle touch, he examined my hands, giving notes to the cowering young doctors. "First, second, and third left digitals slant to the left. First, second, and third right digitals slant to the right. Thumbs normal. Right pinkie bent at first joint. Hand joints raised," he said and then, glancing up from my hands, he looked at me. Was it my imagination or did he agree that my hands didn't match the rest of me?

"You definitely have some damage to your hands and fingers. My first recommendation would be hand molds. We might be able to straighten your slant if you're diligent about wearing the molds. The second alternative is surgery. To straighten your fingers I would first tighten the tendons. For the joints I would make an incision across your knuckles and take down some of the bulging."

I tried to take it all in, my mind racing with thoughts of tied tendons and scars along my hands. "Would they be scarred?"

"The scars would barely be noticeable. I can straighten out the slant and improve the bulbous look of your knuckles. I do one hand at a time. The physical therapy is time consuming, but I know I can make a difference," the doctor said, still holding and studying my hands.

"But would they look normal?" I asked. I couldn't even remember what normal for my hands looked like.

"They would look better. Before you opt for the surgery, let's make molds of your wrist and hands and see what we can do. It's not invasive, you'll sleep in the molds, and we'll know soon if they are going to work."

Overwhelmed with all the information, I nodded. Molds sounded creative and easy. I loved making colorful Jell-O mold salads for the holidays. Who ever thought my latest mold would be of my hands? The young doctors promptly led me to a room where they put my hands, wrists, and arms up to the elbows in a gooey white substance. When they pulled my hands out there was my imprint, slanting to the side. I felt like I was one of the molds at Color Me Mine, soon to be sculptured into a lovely do-it-yourself hand-painted vase.

A few days later I went back to pick up my molds. One of the young doctors greeted me carrying what looked like gigantic arm guards for a hockey goalie, the ones that go all the way down to their giant gloves. They were huge, gray arm sleeves with six heavy black Velcro straps that closed over my hands, leaving the fingertips slightly visible, and covering all of my arms up to the elbow. He strapped me in, and there I stood—robo arms. Not only were they big and heavy, they were bulky, unattractive, and uncomfortable. I looked ready to tackle the first person who came along. So much for the fingerless black lace evening gloves.

"Put them on when you're in bed," he informed me, smiling, pleased at how well they fit.

Sleep, how would I ever be able to get comfortable? Turn over? Hug my husband?

"Wear them every night, and check back with us in a month," he said, removing my robo arms and placing them in a large, white, plastic bag with handles. If they were in a Saks bag everyone would have thought I just bought a new pair of exquisite knee-high boots.

That night, I set my book down and reached under the draped table beside my bed for my hidden plastic bag, pulling my new arm molds up on top of the comforter. Shelly, reading his book, looked over.

"You got your molds," he said, trying not to sound shocked at their hefty size as he watched me fumbling to try to put them on. "Here, I'll help you," he said, pulling the Velcro straps tight on my arms.

I looked down from my sitting position, my arms now covered from fingertips to elbows in my new gear. Two stiff, enormous black Velcro arms in bed with Shelly and me. This would take the romance out of any relationship.

"Yes," I said as I tried to scoot down into a prone position, my arms jutting stiff and straight out on top of the blanket. I tried crossing them, too heavy. I tried turning on my side, but it felt like I had a Velcro-covered plank under my body. I tried bending my arms at the elbow and resting my arms on my chest, not comfortable for anyone with breasts. The only way this would work was if I slept on my back, arms at attention at my sides. There would be no snuggling, no turning over, no restful sleep.

"They're not so bad," Shelly said, trying to make light of my discomfort. "It's better than surgery, Christine. Don't get discouraged."

I closed my eyes, turned my head to one side, and tried to sleep. It was going to be a challenge. And not just sleeping. During the middle of the night I had to take off one of the molds to go to the bathroom and use toilet paper. Oh, the advantages of being a man.

Over the next two weeks I figured out how to sleep uncomfortably, I scheduled sex before putting my robo arms on, and figured out how to maneuver with the bathroom in the middle of the night. My eyes were now even puffier from restless nights, but I was sure my hands were better. Or perhaps they seemed better to me only because my RA pain was worse. How long could I hold out until my Enbrel kit came in? The only medication I was allowed to take was the anti-inflammatory Celebrex, and it just wasn't strong enough. My feet, ankles, knees, wrists, and elbows were grinding away. Bone to bone, what seemed like a gravel pit in my body manufacturing sharp, piercing stones that were wedging their way into my joints, carving out more and more space to pulverize my bones. The only good news was the thought that the stones couldn't break through my skin as long as my robo arms were in place.

"I'm going to schedule the surgery," I told Dr. Kalunian on my next office visit, over a month into my robo arm therapy. "The surgeon was disappointed in the lack of results from the molds. Seems I have stubborn hands." With Dr. Kalunian I was able to let my guard down, shed a tear, take out my frustrations. He never judged me, and always gave his support.

"Think about the surgery, Christine. I have patients who have gone through it and the results, while better, are not perfect. Knowing you, you're looking for perfection. You could be disappointed."

I had heard those words, in a different configuration, from the surgeon as well. Surgery was not going to make my hands normal, just improved.

"Why now, Christine? Why not wait until you see how you do on the Enbrel? Why complicate your life any more than necessary?" Dr. Kalunian asked.

"Because if I can't feel better I need to at least look better. I need to do something to gain some control in my life. What if Enbrel doesn't work? I don't have any other good options. It didn't work on everyone in the research program, I could be one of those patients." I didn't know if it was the desperation in my voice, my damaged hands waving frantically in the air to make my point or the sadness in my eyes that made him nod and say, "Okay, I get it. I need to do some lab work and testing and talk with your surgeon."

I understood that covering up didn't change things. Even in my cocoon of denial I knew that regardless of my own cover-up, I was who I was: that vulnerable little girl who fought for space in the lives of people who mattered. Still, I wanted the surgery.

Covering up wasn't anything new to me. My mom started the cover-up when I was a child. Every time I moved from one boarded house to another my suitcases would be packed and waiting at the door for my mother to come pick me up. My "boarded-out" caregiver and my mom knew I was leaving and moving on, but they never told me. The larger suitcase should have been a clue, because for my sleepovers with my mom I only took a small overnight suitcase. But because it started when I was so young, I never made the connection; large suitcases equals moving day. I grew up in the generation of not talking about anything. Everything was swept under the carpet.

"You don't want to know, Chrissie." "We don't talk about those things, Chrissie." "Why would you even ask about that, Chrissie?" These were the standard answers to my probing questions. Where was my dad? Why couldn't I live with my mom? Why did I have to move to another home?"

To this day when I pack for a trip, whether a business trip or an exciting vacation, as I drive away to the airport and I look at my home there is an ever so slight feeling of anxiety in the

pit of my stomach. Will I see my house again? What if? I have
accepted the fact that I will never be good at leaving.

Over the next week I had every test imaginable to prepare
me for the hand surgery. An echo/ECG for my heart, breathing
tests for my lungs, and coagulating time for my blood. Dr. Kalunian
was not taking any chances. Except for a compromised immune
system, inflamed feet, knees, elbows, and knuckles, I was as healthy
as a farm horse. My hand surgery could be scheduled for the following week. After that, surely the Enbrel would be ready.

Shelly didn't help.

"I don't know why you want to go through with this. You
look perfect to me."

I knew he meant it. To him, the man who didn't acknowl-
edge my weight gain from steroids, pretended that my hands
were normal, and complimented me on my various styles of
sneakers, I was just fine the way I was.

He understood my need for control when I answered,
"Because I have to do something."

Now I understood why my mom would get her comb out
and touch up my hair as soon as we got in the car for one of our
weekends.

"They never part your hair right, Chrissie no matter how much
I tell them," she would say. Turning sideways in the driver's seat
and twisting me to face her, she put the part in the way she liked
it. To me I didn't look any different when she was done but to
my mom I looked like her daughter, not Mama Dorothy's or
Margie's paid houseguest. Was I more lovable? My mom always
seemed to be happier with me when I looked better.

Now I was in a career where my appearance was my calling
card, so presumably the better I looked the more successful, or
lovable, I'd be. The intelligent side of me knew that surgery was a
feeble attempt at control. The emotional side of me accepted my
need for control, however shallow it seemed. I booked the surgery.

The call from UCLA came one morning as I sat in bed watching reruns of *Sex And the City,* trying to eat Doritos (steroid hunger snacks), still in my PJ's, my robo arms back on after Shelly had left for work. If wearing them at night wasn't helping, maybe some additional time during the day would. The only good thing about the morning so far was the realization that it took me longer to get a chip out of the bag and into my mouth. The robo arms diet.

"Am I speaking to Christine Schwab?" the UCLA attendant asked.

"Yes," I answered, quickly trying to swallow a Dorito.

"Your Enbrel kit is ready for pickup."

It's a good thing I wasn't in the room with her; I would have jumped up and hugged her with my robo arms, probably knocking her out cold.

My Enbrel kit, full strength, was ready and waiting. I couldn't get dressed fast enough. Hope, once again, filled my aching joints.

I entered the windowless room No.202 at the UCLA research center, the one room dedicated to patient labs and treatments for those enrolled in research projects. Today I looked at the room differently. Today it was a room of hope, for sure, real hope. For the first time I really noticed the worn Barcalounger chairs, paper towels covering their tattered arms. Metal trays with needles, alcohol, Band-Aids, and cotton balls were ready and waiting. Four white refrigerators were placed around the square room. Each one had sign-up sheets on clipboards hanging on the front and a padlock on the door handle, tightly secured to protect the valuable experimental medicines used in the various programs. The counter held centrifuges, where vials of blood were turning upside down, around and around, to separate and test for levels of disease. Patients of all ages, races, sizes, and genders sat in the various six chairs, some with IVs dripping into their arms. Others filled out questionnaires about their well-being, their pain, their progress or regression. A few with their heads leaned back, eyes closed, waited for the unproven medications to settle in their bodies before they were allowed to leave.

I was now a regular, like Norm on Cheers. I knew the routine. I had practiced my first injections here, my hands shaking as I squeamishly tried to put the needle through the skin of my upper thigh. The sight of blood, needles, and centrifuges no longer intimidated me.

Tina, the technician, took a blue nylon insulated box with handles out of the locked refrigerator and handed it to me. An expensive Hermès alligator bag couldn't have looked as good as this little blue one.

"Here's your kit, same as during the double-blind test. You mark the diary with the date and time of each injection. Note anything that is different or unusual to you. Save the used needles in this red plastic box and return them on your next visit. Keep the medicine refrigerated. If you travel, pack it in ice. If it's not kept cold it will affect the treatment." Tina's demeanor never changed. She had seen the highs and lows of medical testing too many times to let emotion come into the equation. Today her somber facade couldn't diminish my expectations. I walked out carrying my latest and hopefully greatest accessory.

Over the course of my years at UCLA I had left the medical center in many moods. Total depression, total euphoria. In pain and in relief. Accepted and rejected. Today, I left feeling positive. In my new blue plastic bag I held the hope of more control over my health. I no longer thought about the what-ifs; would it work, would I have complications, would I be allergic? I had traveled that road of ups and downs of chronic illness. I had been swollen with steroids, green with nausea, watched my hair fall out from Cytoxan, lived with constant ringing in my ears because of penicillamine and almost died in the hospital from methotrexate. I had hobbled instead of walked, lived with my joints stiffening after any prolonged sitting position, and watched my hands age almost overnight. I had given up hope, but only for short periods. I had to believe I would get better, but it was becoming more difficult. On some days I had even turned my Believe rock over, all hope gone. For more than seven years I had vacillated back and forth between hope and despair, and lately despair held the lead. Uncertainty. My life was uncertain. Even with my desperate grasping for control, control was always outside my reach. Shelly never gave up hope, at least not openly to me. Dr. Kalunian never gave up hope. I wished I could have said the same.

"You're doing amazing. Really, look at you. You're beautiful, nobody would know anything was wrong," Shelly would say every time I dressed for an event. "Beautiful." That's when I knew my denial worked. I could even fool Shelly. But more and more I saw people looking at my hands, watching me slowly rise from a table. Even with my clothes adjustments, my movements were wobbly and deliberate. The fear that my cover-up wasn't working haunted me. How long could I hold onto my career? Who would I be without it?

I felt safer in my marriage. Slanted hands, swollen joints, Shelly didn't seem to care. He had passed the ultimate test. He was staying. If only I could see myself as he did. And I tried. Really, every day I tried to see myself through his eyes but my mom's critical vision always crept in.

"Chrissie, who did your hair for TV this morning?" she would ask me on my routine phone call to her after a national segment. "Did you pick out that dress?" She didn't have to go into details, she could trigger my insecurities with just one question in that special tone in her voice. "I did my hair mom, and that's my favorite new dress," I answered, trying to stand up to her. I sounded strong through the phone but inside my fears of not being good enough, not looking good enough roared, fighting for space inside my RA-riddled body. I wanted to believe Shelly's words, but my mom still had the upper hand.

But now, leaving the UCLA building that had been the focus of my life for more than seven years, I was living two lives. The life of a chronically ill research patient, praying for hope, and the other the life I dreamed of, the career and marriage the movies and books had always promised. I never took my good life for granted. I knew it could go away in a minute, just like my mom always went away in my childhood, regardless of my begging and pleading. But I also knew that the disease could go away at any moment. I could go into remission. I could be normal.

With each step I convinced myself that Enbrel was going to work. Today I thought only about the possibilities. In my strong moments, I always believed anything was possible in life, or at least almost anything. Today I felt these possibilities even in my eroded bones and worn joints and in my slightly broken heart from the expectations and disappointments of too many treatments. I felt it in my soul. It was possible because I had believed it could be possible in the research program. It was possible because I rose above and past my childhood. I survived the insecurities of living with people who didn't care about me. I survived the insecurities of a career where security was not in the equation. I survived because I now had a man who loved me, damage and all. Today, walking toward the UCLA parking structure, seeing the patients all around me, I smiled. I had come to terms with the knowledge that it wasn't what I presented to the outside world that defined who I was, it was who I was inside that mattered. Today I knew I would survive.

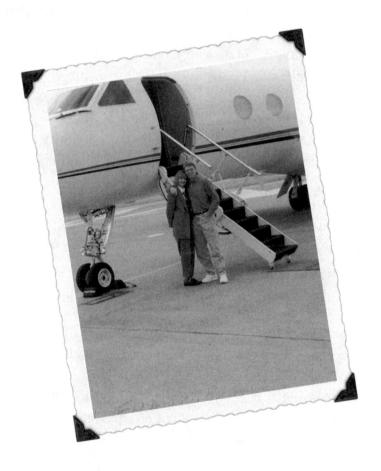

Shelly and I outside the Universal private jet-crop

18

The Enbrel Honeymoon

I closed and locked the door to my bathroom, unzipped my new blue insulated medicine bag, and took out the two needles, one for drawing the water from my purified water bottle and then inserting it into the tiny glass vial with the white Enbrel powder and pink plastic top. The two alcohol cotton squares were wrapped individually. I remembered the first time I injected myself during the double-blind study, thinking it was Enbrel, but later learning it was nothing but purified water. My hands were shaking then as they shook now. The only difference was my hands are now distorted. They don't work like they used to. They don't look like they used to. And I am now medically jaded. I'm a skeptic. I'm a realist. I knew from the test results that some people did well on Enbrel, some got a little relief, and others continued their spiral into arthritic deformation and pain. Part of me was on a high that I had been able to weather the program and was entitled to the drug years before it became available to the public. Another part of me thought, what would be distorted next if this medicine didn't work? How long did I have before my secret was out and my career was over? Fear and hope, fighting for space in my head.

Shelly knew not to bother me when I was doing my injections, especially on this day, the first day of my full-strength Enbrel. He was upbeat and positive. He had planned a two-week vacation to Italy. We had talked and talked about going to Italy and now it was a reality. The travel executive at Universal had made all the arrangements. The trip of a lifetime. Venice, Florence, Rome, and Positano. I needed to feel good. The timing of the start of the full dosage of Enbrel and the trip wasn't exactly perfect because I only had a week of the new Enbrel before we left on the trip. I had now become fearful of not only being too far away from my doctors but also of the complications from starting any new medications. We began planning the trip in April when I had only been in the research program for a few months and thought I was moving toward remission, which later turned out to be just the positive results of stopping all the toxic drugs I had been taking over the years. I didn't know then that I was injecting a placebo into my body instead of any medication. I had no idea that soon the good health I was feeling as the old medications exited my body would soon be replaced by the arthritis army starting their march through my joints all over again.

Now the trip was almost here, and I was starting from square one with a new medication. What if the medicine made me sick like methotrexate? What if I couldn't walk or stand like at the Oscars? What if I ended up in bed, the drugs eating away at my stomach like at the NATPE convention in New Orleans?

Slowly and deliberately I pushed the needle through the skin of my upper thigh and watched the medicine go in as I pressed the plunger down. I could feel the medicine enter my body, slowly, making a raised white area as it lay under the skin, ready to move into my system. There, it was done. My first injection of the real, full-strength Enbrel. I pulled the needle out and looked at it, now empty of all liquid. With my slightly crooked index finger I rubbed the now red injection site, helping the medicine to disperse into my system. The rest was in the hands of who? God? The pharmaceutical company? Or would my own body decide if this drug would work or not? I didn't know, the doctors didn't know, the manufacturers of Enbrel didn't know. That's what research is. I had made the cut to this point. The question remained: How much further could I go? Would I be a good statistic or a failed one? Would I have to start all over with new combinations of my old drugs as I awaited more research drugs or would I be in remission? And why had I ever agreed to go to Italy with all of these unknowns ahead of me?

The next week I visited UCLA for my checkup. They took my blood. I filled out the same questionnaire: How has your health changed over the past week on a scale of one to ten, list all the things you are able to do on your own (buttons, open car doors, open jars), overall rate your health on a percentage chart, one hundred percent being perfect. And then came the release forms, the disclosures. Someone died from cancer, someone committed suicide, someone had a heart attack. Of course, they stated, these things could have occurred without the drug, but they had to inform us, government rules. We had to sign that yes, we knew what had happened and we still wanted to continue in the program. I signed willingly.

"Go on your trip, you'll be fine. I'm a phone call away if you need me. I think this is going to be your drug, Christine. So far you're tolerating it well," Dr. Kalunian told me. He wasn't in charge of my progress anymore. I was under the care of Dr. Bulpitt who was running the research program, but Dr. Kalunian knew me. He knew my history. He understood how hard I had fought to get this far. All the necessary lies I had had to tell and how desperate I was for relief. And in the end, Dr. Kalunian was right. I did just fine. I still packed my sneakers in my suitcase, included pain pills just in case, and took the emergency numbers of all my doctors. For the first time I also included a pair of small heels and a pair of loafers, in the hope that I might be able to squeeze into them. Sneakers just don't look very good with everything, regardless of how creative the outfit.

My first week in Italy was good. My second week in Italy was great. In Italy I carried my blue insulated medical bag as if it were the crown jewels. It became my own personal designer bag. I placed my medicine in the refrigerator at every location. I kept my ice packs to keep the medicine cold during travel in the freezer. By my third week back at home, if it wasn't for the damage in my hands, I was beginning to forget the chronic pain. I didn't have to fake Sparkle Plenty. I was in remission. I was feeling good. No problems, my pain was subsiding, my swollen and inflamed joints were returning to normal. My hands didn't shake anymore as I injected the Enbrel. I couldn't wait to get it into my body. Two shots a week brought me closer and closer to normal. Closer and closer to the life I had lost.

Right after I got back from Italy, I went to UCLA, where my labs were improved. I filled my chart out with high marks in how I evaluated my health, and then Dr. Bulpitt, in his serious and sullen way, gave me the same high marks. Was he afraid to say this drug was working? Would something change during the trial? What did he know that I didn't know? Or was he just sullen while I was ecstatic?

Thinking back, Dr. Bulpitt was always sullen.

19

Nightly and Me

Did I still have rheumatoid arthritis? I would have to pinch myself to remember my pain, my frustration, my seven-year fight with arthritis, because now I was in remission. The only reminder was my slanted hands. I had a full year of pain-free, back-to-normal living. Part of me thought maybe I'd wake up one morning, and the dream would be over, arthritis would be back. Fear still reserved a small space inside my head. Anxiety still could make my stomach rumble. My closet full of sneakers seemed to look up at me when I opened the closet door and say, "We're here, we're ready if you need us." But I didn't. Damage had made my feet still sensitive and four-inch stilettos would never be a part of my style, but I was able to wear low heels, stylish flats, and oxford lace-ups that had gathered dust in my closet over my arthritis years. My feet had grown a full shoe size from damage, and my workout sneakers still required custom-made inserts to take the pressure off where the arthritis had eaten away at the padding on the bottoms of my feet, but overall? I was healthy. I took Celebrex, an anti-inflammatory drug, along with my Enbrel shots, and between the two of them I was pain free. Dr. Kalunian was sure that at some point I would be able to wean off the Celebrex.

Reminders of past pain and difficulty in doing simple things would pop up in my head as I opened a milk carton for the first time and it didn't hurt my fingers, or I would write out a thank-you note without my hands cramping and dropping the pen. And I no longer had to stand up and adjust pretend wrinkles in my clothing in order to get my balance. I popped up like the Energizer Bunny, batteries charged and ready to take off. It's amazing how fast you forget pain. Like childbirth, once the pain is gone, it fades in your memory, because you have the beloved prize of a baby, only this time my beloved prize didn't cry and wake up for two o'clock A.M feedings.

The call came the morning after Thanksgiving. Our home was filled with Shelly's visiting family still sleeping. The holiday table was still decorated, the tablecloth still in place, now stained with gravy and cranberries. The leftovers stacked in their plastic containers and ziplock bags in the refrigerator, waiting to be warmed up for that anticipated lunch, the second turkey feast.

I was awake when the phone rang.

"Christine, it's Magalie, from the Fox morning show. I moved over to *Nightly* and never had a chance to say good-bye. Anyway, today I'm working on a story about the biggest shopping day of the year, and I'd like to use you as the fashion authority."

Because Magalie, my former producer at the New York Fox local morning show was gone when I was there last and nobody seemed to know, or want to tell me, where she had gone, I hadn't talked to her for six months. Poof, the magic television disappearing act. One day you're there, and the next day you're gone and nobody seems to know what happened to you, good, bad, or indifferent. Television is notorious for pretending someone has vanished when they leave for another show.

"What's *Nightly*?" I asked, trying to put the pieces together.

On the other end of the line Magalie cracked up, "*Nightly* is *NBC Nightly News*. I'm a producer here now, and it's the greatest."

The national network news? I have worked on local news, but never national.

Magalie interrupted my thoughts, "I'm doing a story on the day-after- Thanksgiving shopping. Are you available this morning? I know it's late notice, but you know the news business, we always decide on stories at the last minute."

I looked down and realized I was in bed, still in my robe, coffee cup in hand, and the latest copy of *Vogue* open in my lap. My hair hadn't seen a comb since the day before. It was 8:23 A.M.

"I'd need you at the Glendale Galleria at eleven o'clock. You'll hook up with the reporter there. He'll have questions to ask you and basically you take him through some stores and talk about why this is such a huge shopping day," Magalie said.

Glendale Galleria. I was in our new Newport Beach home. Glendale was over an hour away, and I had no idea how to get there. All I knew was I would have to leave by nine thirty to get parked and inside the mall by eleven o'clock. I glanced in my bedroom mirror and looked at the condition of my hair. It wasn't looking like a good hair day.

"Well?" Magalie prodded.

"Sounds great," I answered, taking the phone into my closet to see what I would wear as Magalie filled me in on my contact and the location for the meeting. "We'll turn this around, and it'll be on the evening news tonight."

I was reeling. What to wear? No time to wash and blow out my hair. I had one hour to get myself together, print out driving directions to the mall, and get on the road. I could do this. *NBC Nightly News.* Yes, I could do this. Quickly I ran downstairs to get cottage cheese to coat my stomach for the daily vitamin regime I now must rush to take without breakfast. I grabbed a protein bar to put in my bag for the drive.

"Ohmygod, that is amazing," my stepdaughter Kerry, always the great television publicist, said when I told her the news as she walked up the stairs still waking up. "That is huge, gigantic, amazing." Kerry was a good publicist because she was always overly enthusiastic. "I'll drive you, that way I can drop you off at the mall, park, and then meet up with you." That was the best suggestion I'd had all morning. I could navigate the MapQuest instructions while she drove. I felt some of the pressure subsiding with her kind offer.

I applied a ten-minute facial on my face, now an apple green color as I attempted to blow dry my hair into some sort of order. The masque dried and did its magic, and my hair, as if ordered, fell into place. It turned out to be a good hair day after all. As I looked in the mirror I thought back to the days only a year ago when I had to pull my hair in a ponytail because my shoulders were so inflamed with arthritis I couldn't hold the hair dryer long enough to style my hair. Twenty minutes later, masque off, I sat down at my dressing table and did my makeup. Even my liquid eyeliner went on nicely. Various family members came upstairs to talk about the news and followed me around as I gathered my clothes to dress. "Out, everyone out, I have to get dressed," I said, escorting them through the bedroom door. Their excitement increased my excitement, meanwhile the clock ticked away.

At 9:27 I walked downstairs, looking like a national news reporter. Conservative suit, stylish oblong scarf open at the neck, flat shoes to get me to the mall, designer pumps in my tote for the taping. My fashion statement was oversized earrings, just enough, not too much. It was a fine line to walk between fashion and business. This report was a business report about fashion, and I felt like my outfit was just right. NBC national news, here I come. At nine thirty, Kerry and I were in the car, munching on bananas, heading toward the 405 Freeway to Glendale. Traffic was light. Everyone was still celebrating Thanksgiving, except those of us who were headed to the malls for the biggest shopping day of the year.

The mall parking structure was a maze of cars, all vying for parking spaces. I hopped out of the car and dashed inside to find a mall swarming with energetic shoppers. Kerry would meet up with me at the Gap, our first location. But something was different. Today I wasn't being dropped off close to a store entrance because I couldn't walk, this time it was only about time, not about pain. I stopped for a moment to realize how far I had come on the arthritis scale in the past year. I stopped, in all the craziness of the mall, on this day after Thanksgiving, to be thankful for how fortunate I was.

The reporter, cameraman, and soundman were there and ready. We talked off camera for a few minutes about the story and then we were ready to roll. I slipped out of my flats and into my heels. I forgot about being a chronically ill patient in remission, I forgot about my distorted hands and became a professional reporter. I walked, talked, and gave consumer information as I took the business reporter through several stores. The cameraman and soundman moved right along with us. We did a couple of pickup shots, a little voice-over, and by twelve forty-five we were done.

In the car Kerry gushed about my performance, but she was a gusher. I was always conservative. I never evaluated my performances until I saw them on air. And that day I didn't have to wait long, because everyone was on the road heading toward malls so traffic was crazy. By the time we got home it was almost four o'clock.

At six thirty everyone gathered around the television, the VCR set to record. Like a lot of people in television, I was not a fan of watching myself on TV with other people in the room. I wanted privacy to really watch and scrutinize, to be overly critical. Guests mean well, but they usually talk over the segment and never see the details. I knew I would have to wait until later to watch it for my own personal evaluation, but, as the *Nightly News* music played to the opening, the moment was still exciting.

And there he was, Brian Williams, announcing my segment. My stomach did a flip-flop but this time not from overmedication. My feet were tucked under me on the couch, pain free, and normal size. Eagerly I sat forward as if it would help me see better. On the TV the reporter and I walked side by side, talking about shopping. My hands were purposely hidden in my jacket pockets. I looked like a healthy, normal, fashionable person. I felt like a healthy, normal, fashionable person except for the fact that I was watching myself on the nightly news.

As I walked toward the camera, telling the reporter why stores like the Gap were now selling personal grooming items and perfumes in addition to their jeans and casual clothes, I couldn't help but notice that I was projecting a different image. I was different. I had gained a new confidence. I didn't know if anyone else watching would have noticed any change. I remembered a few years ago when Shelly assured me I looked fine on television when I knew arthritis was changing my appearance, yet today I could see a difference, a positive difference. Arthritis might have ravaged parts of my body, but I had fought back. I might have lost control of my health for a while, but I managed my ability to deal with adversity. I was still the same expert in style and fashion, but now I was also an expert in surviving. The physical damage I so feared was tucked away in my pockets, but I knew it was there. Physically I was not the same. Emotionally I was not the same. I was stronger. I now knew I could survive anything, even arthritis.

In the past there were many times when I thought perhaps I should stop hiding. That it was time to come forward with my secret. But something always held me back. *Not just yet, don't rock the boat.* Now, if someone asked me if I did the right thing by keeping my disease to myself, on this day after Thanksgiving, having watched the national news segment where I looked healthy and walked in heels, without the aid of any steroids or pain medication, my answer would be an unequivocal "yes."

20

Double-Dipping at UCLA

SPRING 2000

Everything in my life was going smoothly. My health, my career, my wonderful marriage, even my secret was still intact. Life was good. But being me, I needed to grow, and education had always been a way for me to grow, so more than a year ago I had decided to enroll at UCLA.

I now attended UCLA for two totally different agendas. One for my body, one for my mind. I was still in the research program for Enbrel, where I had a monthly appointment at the research medical center, where my labs were checked, my joints were tested, and I filled out the medical questionnaires that I had almost memorized after filling them out so many times over the years. The difference being I was marking the forms with answers rating my overall health at ninety percent of good health, ninety-five percent that I felt I could now control my rheumatoid arthritis with medications, and one hundred percent in the category of how pleased I was with my progress. If you compared my questionnaire at the beginning of the program three years earlier you would swear it was another patient. I had come a long way. I was fortunate to be a lab rat, tested and scrutinized as the medical staff monitored the drug for FDA approval.

The other research patients and I were always kept apart, even in the small lab room. No one ever said it, but we understood not to talk to each other. It was almost like electronic invisible dog fences were in place that would shock us if we crossed over the line. We were all confidential files, known by number more than by name. I was CLS#2, ironically there was a CLS#1. I understood that I would never know who that person was, nor would they know anything about me. If I was alone in the room with the technician I still asked how other patients were doing on the drug that was a miracle for me. And if the technician was in a talkative mood they said things like, "Dallas had to quit, the commute was difficult, and they weren't getting enough response to the medication," or, "A couple of problems with San Francisco, but they're staying in the program because they know that once they leave, they'll have to wait until the medicine is FDA approved before they can go back on it." We all understood the strict "take it or leave it" policy. you quit, you were out. Regardless. The same rules applied in the double-blind study, when I had stayed in even though my hands were gnarling and pained. I didn't have any other option. So I understood the severity of the decision when I heard someone had dropped out. They had to be experiencing major complications to give up. You just don't give up hope if there is even a fraction of an ounce left. The doctor still checked my joints, or the monthly "squeeze test" as I liked to call it, even though now it no longer hurt. During the double-blind study, when my joints were inflamed, it was extremely painful. I always wondered if they had to squeeze quite so hard to be able to grade me from one to ten on the inflammation chart. I had learned that even if my joints were visibly inflamed, the "squeeze test" had to be performed, regardless. In order to keep the drugs in research available to UCLA, all lab tests and physical tests had to be inclusive. I had to completely fill out every questionnaire and chart whether I had sore joints or not.

In the lab room I would see patients arriving and leaving, never knowing what drug they were testing. It was obvious some, like me, were doing well, others clearly were declining, but we all were moving medical research forward for future immune-system patients. Basically we were all the same. We had come to a point where our options were exhausted, and it was research or give up. If you were lucky you did well on the new drugs; if you weren't, you declined. Really, none of us had any other alternative except to live a life of pain. And so isolated and alone in our trial treatments, we moved through the halls of UCLA, charts and insulated medicine bags in hand. The progress of medicine. As we passed each other in the halls, we would always sneak a peek, like job candidates vying for a limited number of positions, and make silent health comparisons on the scale of life, trying to figure out just where we fit in.

Simultaneously, at the opposite end of the campus I was a student in the UCLA Extension Writers' Program. With evening and weekend classes, this program allowed me to work in television while I furthered my education. The contrast between the research program and the writers' program was staggering. As a writing student I was taking classes taught by Hollywood legends Garry Marshall *(Pretty Woman, Happy Days)* and Aaron Sorkin *(A Few Good Men, The West Wing, The Social Network)*. Having already published one book on accessories, I was determined to learn more about writing and publish other books.

My teacher Hope Edelman, who wrote the *New York Times* bestseller, 'Motherless Daughters,' inspired me to write a memoir. In her class we heard stories about dysfunctional childhoods, marriages gone bad, murders, and small-town girls making it big. The students were as fascinating as their stories. I soon became a fan of memoir. Certainly I had the childhood for a story. I had the divorce for another, and I was a small-town girl who made it in television. Luckily no murders were involved.

In the extension classroom I was among healthy people immersed in learning. We were free to talk and share with each other and exchange stories, ideas, dreams, and goals. I stopped short of writing about my arthritis; even memoir writers have their secrets. It astonished me how on one campus I could be involved in two totally different areas of education. One educating the medical field and the FDA about new medications, the other educating my mind for new adventures. The lab rat and the student, living side by side at the same university and in the same body.

On this particular day I was writing about my childhood. I had accepted the explanation that because my mother worked she was unable to keep me with her when I was a small child. I believed this because I needed to believe it. Now as I wrote, the truth stared back at me with appalling clarity. Other writers in my class wrote about their single mothers who had babysitters or nannies in order to keep their children at home. Dealing with my own divorce, the thought of my son not living with me never once entered my mind.

Only on my computer screen did the truth come out. My mom was selfish. I didn't want to believe it, but there it was, in black-and-white print, right in front of my eyes. She cared more about her life than mine. I knew the stories about my mother's mother dying when she was only eight, leaving my mother and her twin basically on their own. My mother was one of Hope Edelman's Motherless Mothers. She never had a role model to teach her about being a mother. I could defend her and also say that she was only nineteen when I was born. I could support that with the fact that she had had a hard life, including her marriage to my dad, and all that was valid, but bottom line, I still could have lived with her. Other divorced mothers managed. She could have afforded a nanny, maybe at the exclusion of her new powder-blue convertible and fashionably furnished apartment, but it could have been a possibility. Instead she chose for me to live in other people's homes. The most interesting piece is that as a child I was never angry at my mother. Once I finally got to live with her, at the age of nine when she remarried, I was elated. She was, after all, my beautiful mom.

The pages flowed and with each one came a little more insight into why I was so fearful of losing to RA all I had acquired as an adult. Reading my own childhood pages I saw how insecure I was when it came to my position in life. I knew how fragile my career was and how quickly it could be taken away from me. I realized that all the male figures in my life had left, so why wouldn't Shelly? Arthritis seemed to have the power to take everything away. Being clean and neat with my outfits matching were lessons that served me in my childhood and my career. But when disease struck, arthritis marched over everything, not caring what it destroyed. Not caring if my outfits matched or my hair was parted on the right side. After what I perceived as so many years of making my life perfect, the fear of having it implode overrode any rational thought.

And so the halls of UCLA dominated my life in two very positive ways. Both my mind and my body were being healed at this institution of learning. I was no longer the sick patient, I was the healthy one. I was no longer the confused, insecure little girl. Through many therapy-type discussions with my two insightful half sisters, I had an understanding of who I was and what I had overcome. I had a vague comprehension about why I needed to keep my secret, but now, through my writing, I was beginning to understand that it went much deeper than just fashion and television.

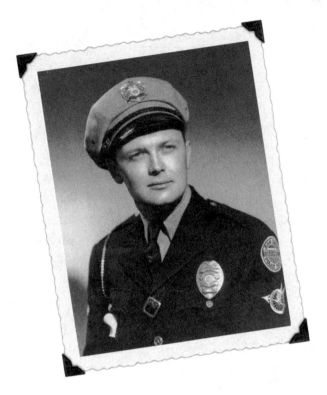

On the surface my parents
looked like the ideal mom
and dad.

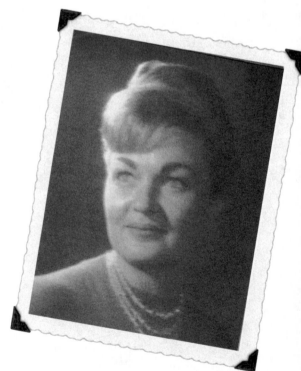

21

This Grown-Up Girl's Osteo Race

OCTOBER 2007

My second book party was at the Façonnable store on Wilshire Boulevard in Beverly Hills with *Vanity Fair* hosting. My book, *The Grown-Up Girl's Guide to Style* was a beautiful oversized hardcover, full of pictures of over-forty women looking fabulous. Earlier that day I spent several hours in my publisher's new Century City offices, signing books that would be given out to the guests that night. My publisher was Judith Regan, the hottest in the business. I was walking—no, running—on cloud nine. Life was not just good, it was great. My rheumatoid arthritis had been in remission for almost ten years. Pain free. My marriage was wonderful, my career at full speed.

My stepdaughter and her husband treated me to hair and makeup for the book launch party. For my outfit I chose gabardine cropped pants, with big side pockets for my hands, black heeled boots, a crisp white shirt, and black velvet jacket. So many friends and coworkers were there, eating, drinking, and congratulating me. A professional photographer covered the room, capturing the celebration with her lens. Music played, wine and champagne flowed, white-jacketed waiters passed hors d'oeuvres, joyous conversations filled the room. Judith Regan was the host of the party, but right before she was to make the opening introduction, Cassie Jones, her number-two person, came over to me.

"Judith's stuck in New York. Sorry she can't make it. I'll be introducing you," she said, trying to make light of it.

It felt like a punch in the stomach. Judith Regan was a celebrity in her own right. When you mentioned her name, people paid attention. She was the queen of publishing, and since her move to Los Angeles, rumored to be expanding her dynasty into all media. Judith and I had had a difficult and long ordeal getting this book in print. Judith liked what was known as "crash books" and one after another they kept getting in the way and delaying mine. A crash book is a celebrity story that breaks in the news, and a publisher decides to get a book out immediately to cash in on the publicity. Judith's latest crash book was OJ Simpson supposedly admitting that he killed his wife, Nicole. It took almost two years for my book to be printed, and then it was printed only because my contract said two years was the limit to either print or return the book to the author. Judith didn't want to lose the book, and so we finally went to press. The roller-coaster ride to publish this book had been difficult, but now I had a book, I had a party, but Judith was a no-show. I kept the smile on my face. I wouldn't let this ruin such an important night. And it didn't. After the initial disappointment I was caught up in the best part of publishing, the celebration of a new book with friends and family.

The publicity tour was intense, just the way an author wants it to be. *The Today Show, LIVE! With Regis & Kelly, CBS Early Show, Entertainment Tonight, Inside Edition*, the *Rachael Ray Show*, and other smaller television and radio shows. *O, The Oprah Magazine* promoted the book by doing a spread on my theories for women over forty dealing with their neck issues. The Associated Press, the *Washington Post Book World*, and The Huffington Post all did stories.

The only reminder I had of my disease was a slight ringing in my ears due to certain earlier medications—it was like having my own internal sound machine—and thinner hair that now required bodybuilding shampoos and lots of thickening spray.

In the midst of all the publicity I had my checkup appointment at UCLA. Dr. Bulpitt had moved on to another medical facility. Dr. Harold Paulus, an elderly icon in the rheumatology department at UCLA, was brought out of retirement to take over the remainder of the Enbrel research program. Because of my many years of steroid use, my bone density had moved into the osteopenia zone, and a year before I'd gone on Fosamex, a weekly pill developed to halt the softening and deterioration of my bones. Despite this medication, I had now moved over to the osteoporosis zone. I was haunted remembering how my mother fell and broke her hip the previous year, was never able to do the rehab after surgery, and never recovered. Dr. Paulus sensed my concerns and put me on Forteo, a daily injection from a penlike instrument containing a tiny needle that dispensed medicine developed to build bone. He also recommended I see a rheumatologist specializing in osteoporosis, Dr. Alan Metzgar, a Beverly Hills physician who treated many celebrities. For the next two years I injected Forteo and watched my bone density numbers improve. My body was actually building bone. The doctor added megadoses of vitamin D, Pilates and Yoga classes, and maximum-strength calcium supplements. I was in a race against brittle bones, and I was determined to win. Proactive had become my mantra.

Eventually, I decided the hand-repair surgery was not for me. I would only get some cosmetic improvement, not enough to justify the invasive surgery. I could do everything I wanted to do with my hands: garden, writing, opening most jars. The only thing I couldn't do was talk with them like I once did and so I continued to hide them as much as possible on television, always looking over my shoulder to see if anyone was watching. Shelly assured me my hands were not that noticeable. I wanted to believe him, but I knew his vision was clouded by love. Spread out in front of me I saw veined, slanted, bulbous jointed hands— not what you want to see on a television fashion reporter.

Toward the end of my mother's life, she was too sick to notice my hands, yet I still knew that they were not her definition of being perfect. But somehow, I was getting used to them. I had let go of the "perfect" and now embraced the "healthy." Perfect didn't mean much when you were really sick. With the distortion of my hands, my priorities had changed. And yet still, I kept my secret intact. I wasn't that secure . . . yet.

The secrets in my family were now in the open. With my dad's passing in 1961, I finally found out where he was for the six years he went missing. He had asked Shelly to go through his files at the very end of his life, and it became obvious that there was a six-year period of files missing. My dad was a meticulous record keeper, so the omission was glaring. And where was his college diploma?

On my next visit to see my mom and my aunt, my sister Pam accompanied Shelly and I. We sat in my mom's living room and talked about my dad, and then I asked the question, "Where was he when I was young?" My aunt and mom both looked down at the floor and frowned. "You don't want to know, Chrissie," they almost said in unison. But I did want to know. I needed to know because somehow in the back of my mind part of his disappearance must have been because of me. I wasn't good enough, he didn't love me enough, or I did something to make him leave. If it wasn't about me, why would he have left me?

Slowly the story came out. My sister Pam wrote it all down on paper, tears streaming down her face. Shelly stared in total disbelief. I tried to take it all in but it was overwhelming. My mom and aunt still stared at the carpet as they talked.

My dad, the man who read mathematical books I couldn't even begin to comprehend, who taught me how to use a slide rule because he wanted me to be an engineer, who made a successful career as an engineer and had many patents for water-saving flow-control devices, had been in prison. Six years of his life behind bars at San Quentin because he stalked my mom and held my aunt hostage at gunpoint. If he were alive his rationale would be that my mom had left him, taking me when she found out about his affairs and he was trying to get her back.

I never knew anyone who was even arrested. My brain heard what was being said, but it was as if they were talking about someone else, a movie. A TV plot, not my dad. We had never been close. How can you be close to someone who is gone from the most formative years of your life?

And sl]owly, over the next month, maybe the next year, the pieces of my shattered childhood puzzle slowly fell in place. The biggest revelation of all was that it wasn't about me. I now knew that my mom's decision to board me out was made based on her needs, not mine. And my dad made his bad choices because he thought he was trying to save a marriage he had previously destroyed. His intelligence was overruled by his passion. Now I understood that my dad didn't take me into consideration when he made his bad choices. It wasn't about me. None of it was really about me, I just happened to be in the way at the time. Overall, the knowledge empowered me because I now knew I wasn't the cause. Still, when all the shock had settled, it mostly made me sad. Sad for what could have been. Sad for the lost childhood. Sad for the minimal relationship I had with my dad. Sad for all the lost years with my mother. I wasn't sad for me, but for all the lost possibilities of how life could have been better.

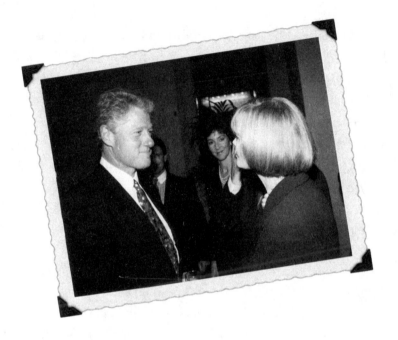

My conversation with President Clinton inspired me to become active.

22

A Makeover for Arthritis?

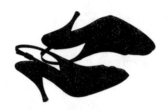

SEPTEMBER 2010

The word arthritis is a sixteenth-century Latin term that came from the Greek words for joint (arthro) and inflammation (itis). For most people, the word conjures up images of the old, crippled, and disfigured—all the words I feared when I heard my diagnosis more than twenty years ago. I had so many misconceptions about the disease, just like so many people still do today.

No wonder. During my twenty-one years living with arthritis and through my research for this book, I've seen mostly pictures of elderly people in hospital gowns with crippled hands and hopeless faces. Even with the pioneering magazine *Arthritis Today* and the Arthritis Foundation making such encouraging headway to forge new, positive images for arthritis sufferers—which they have—book and magazine publishers, the Internet, and advertisers often still use the old stereotypes.

Millions of people suffer from arthritis—the Arthritis Foundation estimates forty-six million people. One in five adults in the United States report having doctor-diagnosed arthritis. According to the Centers for Disease Control and Prevention, an estimated 506 million adults in the United States reported being told by a doctor that they had some form of arthritis, rheumatoid arthritis, gout, lupus, or fibromyalgia. But the reality is that arthritis is no longer a disease that strikes just the elderly. In the past, children, teens, and young adults were misdiagnosed because doctors didn't even consider arthritis as a possibility for these younger patients. Today all that has changed. Children, young adults, and middle-aged people have arthritis. One in every 250 children under the age of eighteen has arthritis.

The other reality is that more and more people are living full, wonderful lives with arthritis. More than fifty percent of rheumatoid arthritis patients are in remission because of research and the testing of new drugs. Fewer patients with osteoarthritis are as well controlled but researchers believe that in the next ten years the percentage of these patients with controlled symptoms will approach the fifty-percent mark they've reached with rheumatoid arthritis.

Arthritis is no longer a life sentence to degeneration, disfigurement, and hopelessness.

So what will it take to make the public aware that there is hope and life for arthritis sufferers? Awareness. Hollywood celebrities have arthritis. Academy Award–winning actors have it. Famous athletes have it. Chart-topping rock stars have it. High-powered politicians have it. And yet, over the years, only a very few minor celebrities have come forward. Of all the diseases, celebrities shy away most from arthritis because of all its negative connotations. Like me, they don't want to be put in that "old and crippled" category. They fear what it could do to their career, to their public perception.

It's human nature. And the question I ask myself is how can we change that perception? How can we give a new face, maybe even a new nickname to arthritis and take it out of the sixteenth century and into the future? Arthritis has changed, but the perception hasn't kept up with the changes. Celebrities—major celebrities—and others need to come forward to put a new face on this disease.

In September 2010 Shelly and I attended the *Stand Up For Cancer* live television show at Sony Studios. My son was working on the production and gifted us with two of the much-coveted tickets to the pre-party, the show, and the after-party. The list of participating celebrities was staggering. More than fifty of the most renowned personalities in TV, film, sports, and music came together to make history. They included George Clooney, Michael Douglas, Jennifer Aniston, Meryl Streep, Lance Armstrong, Halle Berry, Hilary Swank, Forrest Whitaker, Keanu Reeves, Mariah Carey, Beyoncé, Sheryl Crow, Gwyneth Paltrow, and Denzel Washington. The live show was on all the major networks, cable networks, and the Internet and was watched by millions of viewers who donated generously in a tight economy to move research forward. Today it's not only okay to come forward with cancer, it's admired. Celebrities going public with cancer have made a difference not only in raising money for research but also in creating the perception that cancer is no longer a death sentence. You can beat it. There is hope. Meanwhile, arthritis is still shrouded in stigma—stigma that kept me in hiding for more than twenty years.

I remember attending an Arthritis Foundation black tie fifteen years ago honoring one of my close friends. She was the only person, other than my immediate family and my television assistant, who knew about my arthritis. I sat at a table for twelve, my feet throbbing underneath, pain pills ready in my jeweled evening bag. I listened to the incredible stories of the many patients who spoke. There was camaraderie in that room, but I wasn't part of it. I had separated myself, unwilling to publicly join the arthritis group. I looked around at a room of people supporting each other, supporting those suffering my disease, and yet I remained silent. I was the television personality with the top ten "must have" fashion lists, the one who taught people how to put it all together. I believed that hiding my disease was mandatory for my success. Would viewers find my television advice believable if they knew that my own body was falling apart? Pretending to be one thing and actually being another haunted me. I felt guilty.

I was on the outside of where I needed to be. I should have been up there at the podium, sharing my story, doing what I could to help others. But I was afraid. Afraid people would look at me in a different way, no longer accepted into the world of style and television. I was afraid people would see me on Shelly's arm and whisper, "You know, she's almost crippled with arthritis." My issues with abandonment raged inside my inflamed arthritic body. I was afraid my fairy-tale life would go away and I would once again be that frightened little girl vying for her mother's love.

To mask my guilt I gave my financial support to the Arthritis Foundation through my friend. Making donations, buying tickets to events, bidding on items in their silent auctions, taking out ads, and supporting her in fund-raising walks. If I supported the fight against my disease financially, wasn't that doing my part? As a child my mother supported me financially. I always had nice clothes and new black patent Mary Jane shoes. My mother constantly reminded me of how good my boarded-out home care was because they kept me clean and neat. How was I to know that wasn't the definition of a good home? But what about emotionally? Where was my mom? Why couldn't I live with her? Was I, as an adult, now following in her emotionally vacant footsteps? I justified my actions just as my mom justified hers. I was doing the best I could.

But was I?

I had a difficult time even acknowledging that I had rheumatoid arthritis, and I tried not to discuss health, anybody's health, to avoid it. Denial worked for me as a child, and it worked for me when my arthritis flared. The stigma of arthritis kept me in hiding, and I believe it keeps celebrities and others who can make a difference in hiding. One Academy Award–winning actor recently contacted the Arthritis Foundation to be a spokesperson. This actor was ready to come forward. Then their agent found out and talked them out of it.

This person and so many others could be the voices and faces of arthritis, helping to raise awareness and, along with it, money for research. By changing the face of arthritis, we can get more people into remission, take down the pain, and change the arthritis vocabulary. Maybe even have an alternate nickname for arthritis—the Big A. This would be my ultimate makeover. Giving arthritis a new tag, a new look, and its sufferers some renewed hope.

And that's why I'm coming forward now. I want to share with other people whose lives have been changed by arthritis. I want them to go into the remission that has changed my life. I want them to fight, manage their health, and never give up. I want to help.

I hope this book will start that process of changing perceptions and rallying support, but we still need help—a lot of it—and so I urge anyone with arthritis to get involved, to speak out, and to urge others to do the same.

In the meantime, individuals with arthritis will have to go about the business of dealing with their disease. To all of them I would say that what I have learned from life with arthritis is that it is never too late to try to make a difference in your life. Define your disease, but don't let the disease define you. When you're in the middle of pain and frustration, it's easy to give up. The path to wellness is paved with trial and error, and after many trials and many complications sometimes you feel like you can't take even one more. You've had it. I understand. I've been there. Discouraged, too many medications unsuccessfully fighting their own battle inside my body. I wondered how I could fight the battle of arthritis and of medications, and at times I thought I couldn't. I was out of energy. Out of hope.

And it's okay to give up for a day, maybe even two, but then you have to get going again. Giving up is giving in to the disease, and arthritis is a disease that will take over if you give in. It's greedy, it likes to take control, and it wants to win. But you can't let it win.

When I was ready to give up, there were no new drugs, just different combinations of the old drugs. Only Dr. Kalunian's promise of new drugs coming down the research pipeline offered any hope. Today there are many new FDA approved drugs: Remicade, Humira, Orencia, Rituxan, Cimzia, Simponi, and Actemra. Several other new drugs are now in test trials. A few are intravenous, others are subcutaneous—injections like Enbrel. There are options.

I have a cousin who suffers from arthritis. She says her pain is constant. She has tried many things, Enbrel being one of them, and all have failed. When I gave her this list of new drugs I found in doing my research for this book, her answer was, "I won't do any IV. I'm tired of trying new drugs," and so she goes to her doctor every other month for a cortisone shot, which gives her a little relief, but only a little. I equate her treatment to using a Band-Aid on something that needs stitches. Meanwhile arthritis controls her body, damaging, taking control, and winning.

None of us like needles, none of us want to depend on a monthly IV infusion or a weekly self-injected shot, but what is the alternative? I have been afraid of needles since the time I stood in line in elementary school, shakily holding the shot permission slip my foster mom signed that morning, hearing the kids in front of me cry as they were given the shots for polio. Some watched the needles go into the arms of the kids in front of them. I stared at the floor, thinking at any minute I would faint and almost wishing I could so I wouldn't have to get the shot. When I think back about that time I am amazed at the cruelty of lining young children up for shots. No loving parent to hold onto them, no friendly family doctor who knew them, and no closed door to keep frightened eyes from watching. Only a nurse with an alcohol cotton ball and a needle, quickly moving the long line along.

So when I realized I would have to administer my Enbrel with a shot, my elementary school fears came back. I couldn't even watch somebody get a shot. As an adult I pleaded with doctors to avoid shots. How would I ever be able to stick a needle into myself? And this is where we must weigh the options. Hope in a needle vs. no hope. And slowly, fearfully and somewhat disbelieving, I learned to give myself a shot. Now I do it without thinking. I could give others shots if I needed to. I shelved my fears because the results outweigh everything.

Just like so many things in life, finding and maintaining good health can be full of trade-offs.

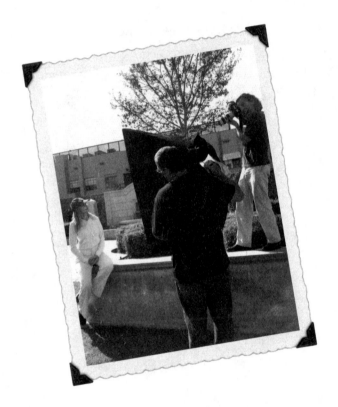

Today I feel I am back to who I used to be.

23

The Future

After more than eleven years of collecting patient data, the Enbrel research program at UCLA closed in May 2010. Eleven years of questionnaires and charts went back to Amgen, the parent company of Enbrel, and all the patients returned to the original rheumatologists they saw before the program began. The FDA had approved Enbrel for public use in 1998, and the patients who stayed in the research program after that were the long-timers, the ones who had weathered the ups and downs— patients like me, who had good results. We were the postmarketing, open-label extension study that had completed the long experience safety data the company required. Now we needed to move on in order to make room in the research center, especially in the Barcalounger chairs, for future drug-testing patients.

My feelings about seeing the program close were mixed. On one hand I was delighted to be in such good health that I no longer needed UCLA. On the other hand, UCLA had been my second home. I spent nineteen years of my life as a patient there— eight in the 200 Medical Center building and eleven in the research department. Nineteen years of my life with arthritis. And UCLA was where I went when I was desperate and an IV infusion of steroids could put me back on track. The place where

I knew everyone and they knew me on a first-name basis. The halls where, regardless of my condition, I felt healthy compared to so many patients who were much sicker than I was.

So when I walked out of the UCLA research building for the last time I no longer noticed the peeling paint, the worn linoleum, or the outdated magazines in waiting rooms where patients sat for hours, hoping for miracles. The UCLA Medical Center represented the place where hope finally materialized for me. UCLA had been like a good foster home. I wished I didn't have to be there, but when it came to moving out I almost didn't want to leave, the fear of the unknown looming close by.

Dr. Kalunian moved to the University of California at San Diego, the Center for Innovative Therapy, to continue and advance his work as a professor of medicine in the division of rheumatology and immunology. When he first left UCLA I felt as if I had lost my support system, but being the doctor he was, I quickly found out that he would always be there for me. He was the person who kept me going through the darkest days and nights of my disease. He never gave up on hope, or me. And time after time, he rescued me, eventually directing me to the research program that changed my health. What do you say to someone who gives you your life back?

I moved to Dr. Allan Metzger, my new rheumatologist, primarily to monitor my osteoporosis. My rheumatoid arthritis no longer needed much oversight. With my weekly Enbrel shot, I remained in the world of the healthy. I had long since packed up my extensive wardrobe of designer sneakers and donated them to charity. I often wondered if any other arthritic feet were filling my shoes. The only sneakers I needed now were for power walking, fitted with individually molded inserts to keep pressure off the areas of my feet where bone had been eaten away when my disease was active. I could walk and walk and walk and all I got was tired. No more inflamed red feet, no more aching joints, no more pain. I was whole.

I have been humbled by arthritis. It took away a lot of my self-esteem. I look at my hands in disbelief. They stare back at me, reminding me that I am not perfect. Over time they have taught me that perfection was not what should be important in life. Do I wish my hands were not misshapen? Of course, I was raised to believe that perfection was what I had to strive for. I am the sum of my superficial and unstable upbringing. No amount of therapy or illness can totally alter those embedded principles from my mind, but arthritis sure changed them. I left behind any trace of arrogance when I walk through the doors of the medical center. When you're a patient, it doesn't matter if you arrive in a chauffeur-driven limousine or on a public bus. It doesn't matter if you are a CEO of a Fortune 500 company or a member of its cleaning staff. It doesn't matter if you look as if you work out every day or if you haven't seen the inside of a gym since high school. Inside, our bodies are diseased. Stripped of our clothes and dressed in hospital gowns, we are all the same.

Disease leaves you desperate for control at a time when you have virtually none. Still, I believe you have to fight back. What I know for sure is that what you can't control, you can manage. You need to be involved in your medical care. It's not about having a lot of money or power, it's about being proactive, being concerned, and finding out what works for you. Your health can't afford for you to take no for an answer. In my lowest moments, when I went for a second opinion to Dr. Wallace, he said that because of all the drugs that had failed me there wasn't much he could do. Yet, the doctor that gave me my initial diagnosis, Dr. Kalunian, never told me that. He always had an answer, a new combination, a new hope. I couldn't always be as positive, yet after I would indulge in my own pity, I would grasp on to his hope and keep fighting. I believe there is a Dr. Kalunian out there for everyone.

I am inspired by heroes like Michael J. Fox and Melissa Etheridge. They deal with devastating health issues and they never give up. They don't shy away from the public, they embrace them. They use their disease to make others aware. My issues seem trivial in comparison and yet to anyone who suffers from any chronic disease or disability, health is never insignificant.

Arthritis has changed me physically, mentally, and emotionally. Physically, my hands are slanted and knobby. Will I ever talk with my hands again? Probably not. I am still vain.

Mentally, I am aware of the importance of good health. We all talk and write about it, and yet it takes something life altering to make us really value our health.

Emotionally, I have more empathy. I see a person with a walker or a cane in a store and I stop to help them. I no longer avoid friends and family with diseases. I recognize that just because it's not pleasant to talk about it doesn't mean it should be ignored. It's not about me. It's about them. I now understand that I have to concentrate on the people who suffer.

After an incredible career in the worlds of television and fashion it is now time to switch gears. My ideal television segment will no longer be filled with beautiful models in designer clothes. Instead it will be talking with a host in a warm and candid manner about real people living with a chronic disease. Will I still be looking over my shoulder to see if anyone's watching? Most likely. I will always feel damaged. The difference is that damage has now created a passion in me to share my story and make a difference. That damage has inspired me, driven me to now talk about my journey.

What I have learned on this journey with health no longer makes me feel the need to run to the stores to change my outsides with the latest fashion must-have. It has made me reflect on what is important in life and changed me on the inside, where it matters. A totally new type of makeover for this twenty-five-year fashion maven.

I no longer feel the need to wear the latest designer shoes. I still appreciate them, but they've lost some of their importance to me. I survived arthritis wearing sneakers. My teaching and sharing now focus on living with a chronic disease. I want others to know that we can all rise above where we come from and take control of where we want to be. Even though at times things might seem impossible, we can overcome what may feel insurmountable if we always look to the future. My passion is to show the path to wellness, how to live with arthritis, the new way. Today with arthritis, almost anything and everything is possible.

I am living proof.

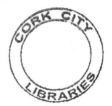

ABOUT THE AUTHOR

Christine Schwab is one of the most successful television personalities and authors in fashion, beauty and lifestyle. She has been a recurring guest on the most popular network television shows including: **Oprah!, NBC Nightly News, CBS–The Early Show, The Today Show, Live with Regis and Kelly, Entertainment Tonight, The Insider, Rachael Ray, Inside Edition, CNBC News, Fox Network News, E! Entertainment, and Weekend Today.**

Schwab started her career as a journalist on **KABC Talk Radio** and **KABC-TV Eyewitness News** in Los Angeles, and became a familiar face in California as a fashion reporter on **ABC'S AM Los Angeles** and **ABC'S AM San Francisco,** where she also served as guest host.

Her most recent book, *THE GROWN-UP GIRL'S GUIDE TO STYLE,* was published in September 2006 by Harper Collins. Christine's first book, *QUICKSTYLE,* was published under her maiden name, Christine Kunzelman, by Random House in September of 1994.

As the contributing style editor to *Redbook* magazine Christine wrote a highly rated monthly column that also appeared in the Australian magazine *She.* Schwab has also been featured in *O, The Oprah Magazine; Newsweek; Vanity Fair; Ladies Home Journal; Women's World; The Chicago Tribune; The Huffington Post; and The Washington Post Book Magazine/Sunday.*

Schwab has also been a spokesperson for many of the country's leading fashion and beauty companies. *Estée Lauder, Revlon, Cotton Inc., Lenscrafters, Patek Phillipe, and The Platinum Guilde* are just a few of the companies Christine has worked with. Some of her private style consultation clients have included: *ABC, Disney, Universal Studios,* and *WABC-TV.*

Christine is a member of Aftra, Fashion Group, Writer's Market, and Pen USA.

ACKNOWLEDGEMENTS

To my agent Carol Mann for always believing in me. We have been through many "publishing adventures" together and I know there will be many more. I thank you for your continued encouragement and support.

To Ann Treistman, Senior Editor at Skyhorse Publishing, for her enthusiasm for my book and for being such a total delight to work with. And to Skyhorse publicist Esther Bochner for her wonderful energy. She defines a good publicist.

To my sister Pam Everett, truly the biggest supporter of this book from it's inception. She kept me going through writer's block and made me dig deeper through the painful times. Thank you for always making me move forward with my story and for being my personal editor. This book wouldn't have been as complete without you. You combine the professor with being the sister, all with love.

To my extraordinary writers group: Hope Edelman, who put us all together, Liz Berman, Amy Friedman, Deborah Lott, and Amy Wallen. This group of brilliant women nourishes me as a writer. Thank you for helping me understand and come to terms with my childhood through writing. To Monica Holloway for being the perfect example of giving back and helping me navigate my way to the Arthritis Foundation.

To the National Arthritis Foundation for their support of this book from the very beginning. John Klippel, President and CEO for understanding my passion. To Debra Neuman, Marcy O'Koon, Carol Galbrea, Hope Cristol, Susan Siracusa, and Kevin Garrett for continuing that support through the publishing journey. I look forward to working with all of you for many years to come.

A special thank you to my sister Susan Whittaker and my children, Erik, Kyle, and Kerry for their support, strength, and encouragement during the difficult years of dealing with Rheumatoid Arthritis. Also thanks to my son-in-law Eric and my Princeton family; Kevin, Dina, Spencer, and Ashley.

To my writing mentor and friend Phyllis Melhado. You offer honest praise and criticism and keep me on the writing path. You celebrate my good days and help me through my tough ones. We are truly writing soul mates.

For the people who have set the bar for being first class in the world of entertainment, Kathie Lee Gifford, Adam Glassman, Terry Goulder, Audrey Kolina, Deborah Norville, and Bonnie Tiegel. I appreciate you!

To those friends who read my pages and give notes along the journey, Marti & John Daly, Ghena Glijansky, Bill Kelly, Judie Jacquemin, Linda Michaels, Julia Serebrinski, Dale Sessa, and Pam Welch. Every writer needs a positive support group of readers and I have one of the best.

For others involved in my book process, thank you to Dr. Harold Paulus at UCLA for his cooperation in tracking down the many years of medical files needed for my research; to Dr. Alan Metzgar for teaching me that Osteoporosis can move backward instead of only forward; LeAnna Weller Smith for designing a stylist unique cover; and to my photographer Rich Marchewka for his beautiful work on both the book cover and my author photos.

A special appreciation to the friends who always show interest in my writing projects, Barbara and Ave Butensky, Pat and Andy Friendly, Jackie Clarkson, George Ann Dennis, Bonny Dore, Steve Hanselman, Bob Jacquemin, Zov Karamardian, Jean and Haig Kelegian, Georgi and Alan Kolsky, Bonnie and Bob Konigsberg, RogerLefkon, Doris & Mick Miguelez, Carol & Buddy Morra, Pam Nicholes, Sandy & Daryl Phillips, Joanne Saltzman, Marc Shatz, Bunny & Mel Shaw, Jimmy Stevens, Cindy Wall, Joanne Weeks, Mark Whittaker,and Carol Weisman.

And finally to my husband Shelly Schwab for making every day an adventure in this special life we share. You encourage me to pursue my dreams in writing. You are my dream in life.